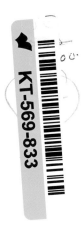

Charcot-Marie-Tooth Disease:
A Practical Guide

also known as
hereditary motor and sensory neuropathy and
peroneal muscular atrophy

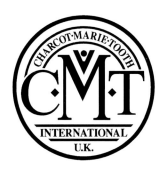

Charcot-Marie-Tooth Disease:
A Practical Guide

also known as

hereditary motor and sensory neuropathy and
peroneal muscular atrophy

Compiled by CMT International UK

First published in book form September 2000

by CMT International UK

ISBN 0–9533883–0–1

Edited by Andrew Northern

Designed and produced by Ray Hadlow FCSD and Jane Hadlow

Typeset in ITC Zapf Book by DP Press, Sevenoaks, Kent

Printed by Saunders and Williams Printers Ltd, Sutton, Surrey

All correspondence and enquiries should be sent to:
The Secretary, CMT International UK, 121 Lavernock Road, Penarth,
South Wales CF64 3QG. Telephone/Fax: 029 2070 9537
E-mail: mereadcmt@aol.com

CMT International UK is a registered charity, number 327971

Disclaimer

While every effort has been made to ensure the accuracy of this publication, CMT International UK cannot accept responsibility for any errors, omissions, misstatements or mistakes, or for any action resulting from its use. The advice given in this book is for general guidance only and is intended to supplement professional medical advice, not replace it. People with CMT should always seek advice from a suitably qualified professional when dealing with specific situations.

Dedication

This book is dedicated to the memory of Professor Anita Harding, professor of clinical neurology at the Institute of Neurology in London, who did a great deal to further our knowledge of Charcot-Marie-Tooth disease. Professor Harding died in 1995.

Preface

Coping with any medical condition for life is a daunting prospect, but it is far more difficult if there is little information about it and even doctors themselves find it hard to diagnose.

This is the problem faced by many people with Charcot-Marie-Tooth disease. It may be the most common inherited neurological disorder, but learning to deal with it often means a long search for answers and help.

We hope this book will change all that. It is a guide for doctors and for those who have CMT. It aims to give fresh insight into the condition as well as plenty of positive advice about how to live with it.

The book is the result of many months of hard work by members of the CMT support group in the UK, many of whom know from their own experiences of coping with the condition how useful it will be. It is a testament to their dedication and inspiration and a valuable legacy for current and future generations of people with the disease.

Julie Etchingham
Patron
CMT International UK

Foreword

In 1886 two French neurologists, Jean-Martin Charcot and Pierre Marie, and an English neurologist, Howard Henry Tooth, described a set of characteristic physical symptoms to which their names were later given: Charcot-Marie-Tooth disease (CMT).

CMT causes a deterioration of the peripheral nerves which control sensory information and muscle function in the hands, forearms, lower legs and feet. This can lead to foot bone abnormalities such as high arches and hammer toes, foot-drop walking gait, scoliosis (curvature of the spine), muscle cramping, problems with balance and hand function, and the loss of some normal reflexes.

It can produce chronic pain and fatigue, and in rare instances it may cause severe disability, but it is **not** life-threatening and it does **not** affect life expectancy.

CMT is not a disease like HIV, for example, or hepatitis; it cannot be 'caught' from another person. It is an inherited genetic disorder which is passed on from parents to children, usually in an autosomal dominant pattern, which means that if one parent has CMT there is a 50 per cent chance of passing it on to each child (though it can vary greatly in its severity even within the same family). There is no wholly effective treatment but some of the effects may be corrected surgically, and physiotherapy, occupational therapy and moderate physical activity have also been found to be beneficial.

Despite being the most common inherited neurological disease in the world – it affects approximately 1 in 2500 of the global population – CMT is still not widely understood. Many medical practitioners do not know much about it and diagnosis is often difficult. A common response is for a doctor to tell a person with CMT that there is nothing that can be done for them and to just go home and put up with it.

While it is true that there is no cure for CMT – at the moment – there are many things that someone with the condition can do to improve their quality of life. With the assistance of sympathetic doctors and other professionals and support from groups like CMT International UK it is possible to lead a good, productive and happy life.

Reading this book is a good place to start. It has been compiled to help people who have CMT, their carers, and medical practitioners who may not be familiar with the condition. It provides a great deal of practical day-to-day advice for living with CMT, much of it based on first-hand experience, but it should not be used as a substitute for professional counselling.

Contents

List of plates and figures

Introduction

Charcot-Marie-Tooth disease is one of a group of superficially similar conditions known as hereditary motor and sensory neuropathies (HMSNs) which cause weakness and wasting of the muscles, especially the muscles in the lower legs and feet and the forearms and hands, because certain nerves do not function properly. HMSNs are inherited disorders which are passed on from generation to generation within the same family. The term refers to the two types of nerves which are affected: motor (movement) and sensory (feeling). A neuropathy is any condition in which nerves are involved.

CMT is sometimes also referred to as peroneal muscular atrophy (PMA) because one of the muscles which wastes away as a result of the condition is the peroneus (the shin muscle).

In discussing the condition some doctors and other health professionals may use the term HMSN while others may call it PMA, but throughout this book it is referred to consistently as CMT.

Part 1
Genetic and medical issues

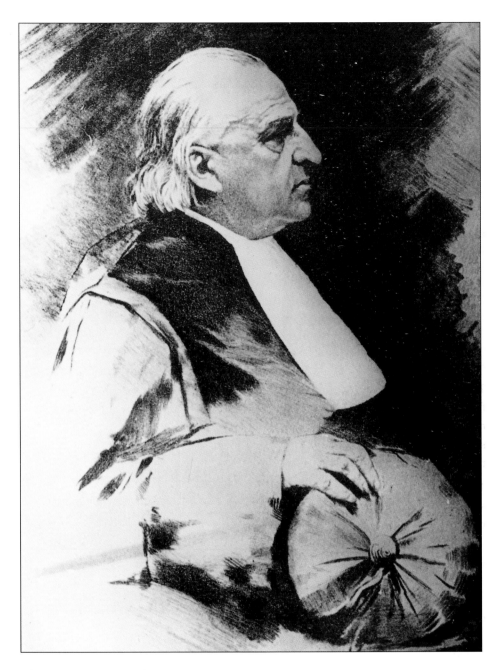

Plate I Jean-Martin Charcot

The causes and symptoms of CMT

CMT affects the peripheral nerves – the nerves connecting the spinal cord to the muscles and joints – which carry electrical messages to and from the brain.

The peripheral nerves consist of two types of nerve fibres: motor nerves, which control movement, and sensory nerves, which permit feeling. The motor nerves and sensory nerves work together like a two-way cable system. Messages from the brain travel via the upper motor neurones, down the spinal cord, through the lower motor neurones (such as the sciatic nerve in the leg) to the muscles. In the sensory system the messages travel the other way: from the sensory neurones to the spinal cord to the brain. If any of these nerves are damaged or defective, as they are in CMT, a person may experience a combination of motor symptoms, such as a weakness or wasting in the muscles in the lower leg, and sensory symptoms, such as numbness or a lack of feeling in the hands and feet.

The peripheral nerves themselves may be likened to electrical cables with an inner fibre, the *axon*,[1] wrapped in a protective insulating sheath of a substance called *myelin*. If the myelin is damaged the nerve impulses tend to be conducted more slowly than usual, whereas if the axons are damaged the speed of conduction is normal but the strength of the signal is reduced.

The effects of CMT can vary enormously in severity even within members of the same family. Usually though, the symptoms are **not** severely disabling and often do not change a great deal after a person has finished growing, although technically speaking they are progressive.[2] It is also possible to carry the *genetic disorder* which causes CMT yet display no symptoms – indeed, between 10–20 per cent of all affected individuals have no symptoms whatsoever – but the risk to succeeding generations remains. (For more about *genetics* and the way CMT is inherited see page 22.)

---

1 Words in italic type are listed in the glossary of scientific and medical terms on page 38.

2 The word 'progressive' is used far too loosely by some less knowledgeable doctors and is guaranteed to inspire panic. To many people the word is synonymous with rapid deterioration, but in the case of CMT it usually means a very gradual loss of strength or dexterity over many years. So while CMT is technically progressive, a person who is diagnosed early in life and shows mild symptoms is **highly unlikely** to deteriorate dramatically during the course of their life.

Generally speaking, the first evidence of CMT is usually detectable between the ages of 5 and 15. It tends to become particularly noticeable at puberty when there is a sudden increase in growth, though sometimes it may not be seen until very much later, even into middle-age.

It is very common for people with CMT – and especially for those with CMT type 1 (see page 16) – to have high arched feet and curled or 'hammer' toes (conversely, abnormally flat feet can also be a problem) and this may be obvious from a very early age. Also, the legs may take on a characteristic shape known as an 'inverted champagne bottle leg': ie, a thin lower leg due to muscle wastage but with a normal thigh muscle's bulk.

This is usually accompanied by a slight difficulty in walking, which is caused by problems picking up the front of the foot. To avoid tripping, people with CMT often raise the knee when walking, resulting in a characteristic 'high stepping' gait.[3] The stresses and strains of walking in this way can be very painful and twisted ankles and sprains are common. (It is worth noting that people with CMT often have difficulty in obtaining comfortable shoes and this can cause additional problems with corns and calluses – see 'Care of the feet', page 54.)

It is **very rare** for people with CMT to lose the ability to walk completely; however, aids such as walking sticks or *orthoses* may be needed in later life, and in very rare cases a wheelchair may be necessary. (For more about orthoses see page 68.)

Another characteristic symptom of CMT is a burning or stabbing pain in the legs caused by the damaged nerves themselves. Leg cramping and 'restless leg syndrome', where the leg muscles feel jumpy, particularly when they are tired, is also common.

Weakness of the hands also occurs in most people but not usually until after the age of 20 (the feet are almost always affected first). A classic 'CMT hand' tends to

---

3   For every muscle that does a particular job there is one which does precisely the opposite. These muscles are called antagonists. Difficulties can arise when one of a pair of antagonists stops functioning; the muscle that continues to function no longer has its controlling partner and this allows changes to take place. The changes that are characteristic of CMT amount to a shortening of the still functioning muscles, which results in changes to the alignment of the lower part of the leg. This is further complicated by the fact that the body is very adaptable and if one muscle stops working another will try to do the work – ie, a muscle not designed for a specific job will make its best effort to do it. So, one non-functioning antagonist leads to shortening in its equal and opposite twin and another muscle will try to do the work of the non-functioning muscle. The shortened muscle pulls the foot inwards from the back of the heel and the 'hard working' muscle, in attempting to lift the foot up, causes clawing of the toes and a very high arch to form in the foot. See also 'Some commonly asked questions about orthotics' on page 68.

have hollows where there should be muscle bulk: ie, at the base of the thumb and between the tendons on the back of the hand. As the muscles which allow the fingers to straighten atrophy, the stronger palm muscles pull the fingers into a fist and the hand takes on the characteristic 'claw' shape. This can make fine manipulatory tasks like writing or fastening buttons difficult.

It is usually the case with both the hands and the feet that there is some degree of sensory loss or numbness (cold feet are especially common due to poor circulation in the lower legs). Very rarely the numbness can be severe and may lead to self-inflicted injuries without the person realising it: burns to the hands from hot cups and ulcers caused by poorly fitting shoes are typical examples. The normal reflexes such as the knee jerk are commonly lost, particularly in CMT type 1, and this is often one of the first signs noticed by doctors. A few people with type 1 also have shaking hands (tremors). This combination is sometimes referred to as the Roussy-Levy syndrome.

There are more complex forms of CMT in which the neuropathy is combined with other problems such as deafness, visual impairment, vocal cord paralysis and breathing difficulties but these are all very rare. Mild curvature of the spine occurs in some people and tends to be more severe in those who have problems with their limbs from an early age.

The different types of CMT

CMT is caused by a genetic disorder – a defect or change in the genetic make-up of the body. Traditionally the commonest forms of CMT have been divided into two main types: type 1, in which the electrical conduction in the nerves is slow, and type 2, in which the nerve fibres are defective.[4] There are many other types of CMT but they are much rarer.

The four most common types of CMT have a number of variations, each of which is described below.

CMT type 1

Type 1 is caused by a defect in the insulating sheath – the myelin – which covers the peripheral nerve fibres in the arms and legs. Normal myelin helps the nerves to transmit messages from the brain very quickly over long distances in the body. If the myelin is damaged the messages are transmitted much more slowly. The technical name for a condition caused by defective myelin is a demyelinating (or hypertrophic) neuropathy.

The age of onset of all variants of type 1 is usually between 5 and 15 years of age although it can start earlier or later.

Variants: type 1a, type 1b, type 1c and X-linked CMT

Type 1a is usually caused by a duplication of a *gene* on *chromosome* 22. Less commonly there is only one gene on each chromosome 22 but one of them is defective. This causes exactly the same symptoms as a duplication.

The gene in question produces a *protein* called peripheral myelin protein-22 (PMP22) but precisely what this protein does in the myelin is not yet known. About three-quarters of all people with type 1 have type 1a, which is detectable by a blood test.

---

4   Scientists now know that different abnormalities in the various genes responsible for the formation of myelin do not always cause a slowing down in nerve conduction. Some people previously categorised as having type 2 on the basis of an electrical test are now known to have a myelin problem.

Type 1b is caused by a defect in a gene on chromosome 1. This gene produces a protein called myelin protein zero (MP0) which is also part of the myelin sheath. Like PMP22 its precise function is not yet known. Type 1b is also detectable by a blood test.

Type 1c is also a demyelinating neuropathy but its genetic origin is as yet unknown. Unlike the other type 1 variants it cannot be detected by a blood test; other methods have to be used, and these are described on page 19.

X-linked CMT is so called because the genetic defect which causes it lies on the X chromosome, one of the *sex chromosomes*. The affected gene produces a protein called connexin 32 which is involved in the formation of channels ('gap junctions') between *cells*. Just how this causes CMT is not yet understood.

X-linked is the second most common form of CMT, accounting for 10–15 per cent of all cases. If a mother carrying an X-linked disorder has children, each of her sons has a 50 per cent chance of developing the disease. Daughters have a 50 per cent chance of being a *carrier*, in which case they could be mildly affected. (For more about the inheritance patterns of CMT see page 22.) X-linked CMT is detectable by a blood test.

CMT type 2

In type 2 the fault lies in the core of the nerve (the axon). The effects are similar to type 1 – ie, messages from the brain are transmitted more slowly, though not quite so slowly as with type 1 – and there are other irregularities in the way the nerves function. Type 2 is much rarer than type 1 and generally develops much later in childhood, typically between the ages of 10 and 20. The technical name for a condition caused by a defective axon is an axonal (or neuronal) neuropathy.

No type 2 variant can be detected by a blood test. Other methods have to be used, and these are described on page 19.[5]

Variants: type 2a, type 2b, type 2c and type 2d

Type 2a is similar to type 1 but the genetic defect is on chromosome 1.

Type 2b is characterised by severe ulceration problems. The defect is on chromosome 3.

---

5   For types 2 and 4 the chromosomal location of some forms is known but the genes have not yet been identified and cannot be tested for in the laboratory.

Type 2c affects the vocal cords and diaphragm. Its genetic origin is unknown.

Type 2d is also similar to type 1. The defect is on chromosome 7.

CMT type 3 and type 4

Type 3 is also known as Dejerine-Sottas disease. It is a particularly severe variant of type 1. The effects are first seen in early childhood.

Type 4 is actually a group of types which can be either axonal or demyelinating. It is mainly confined to ethnic groups in which marriage within the same family is common.

Types 3 and 4 are diagnosed in the same way as type 2.

How CMT is diagnosed

It is very important to establish exactly which type of CMT a person has, especially if they are thinking of starting a family, since any advice given by a *genetic counsellor* will vary depending on the type of CMT and its mode of inheritance. This may require detailed family investigations as some mildly affected family members may not have any symptoms.

In recent years rapid progress has been made in identifying the genetic defects underlying the different types of CMT and it is now possible to test for **some** of these in the laboratory (there is, as yet, no comprehensive genetic classification). This sort of assessment also serves to distinguish CMT from other non-genetic causes of neuropathy, and this is particularly important in people who do not have any affected relatives.

At present CMT type 1a, type 1b and X-linked can be detected by a blood test.[6] Diagnosis of all other types and variants is usually based on a physical examination, including tests of muscle function and sensory response, and nerve conduction studies which measure the speed of conduction of the nerves and the size of the electrical response.[7]

A thorough family medical history is taken to determine whether or not the disorder is inherited (see 'How CMT is inherited', below). In some cases a nerve or muscle *biopsy* may be used to confirm the diagnosis, especially when symptoms are very mild and the family history of the disease is unclear.

---

6   There is a difference between what is theoretically possible and what is currently available in NHS laboratories. Testing is widely available for type 1a, and many laboratories can test for X-linked, but testing for type 1b can only be done at the University of Aberdeen. In practical terms a precise label is not always of great importance with respect to diagnosis, prognosis or genetic counselling – which is in part why tests for the rarer forms are not yet widely available.

7   Over the next few years blood tests will gradually replace electrical tests, which are less reliable. However, electrical tests are still a valuable tool in diagnosing those disorders which cause a marked slowing of nerve conduction. Affected children show the typical electrical abnormality from about the age of 5.

Prenatal testing for CMT type 1a

A person with CMT type 1a has a 50 per cent chance of passing on the condition to each of their children (see the detailed explanation on page 23). Before considering *prenatal* testing – preferably in advance of the pregnancy itself – it is essential to confirm that one of the prospective parents has the duplicated chromosome 17. There is no point in testing for the duplication in families who have other types of CMT.

The prenatal test is done by *chorionic villus sampling*, which involves taking a sample with a fine cannula through the neck of the womb, usually in the tenth week of the pregnancy. It can be done later than the tenth week, but if the pregnancy is terminated it is much more unpleasant for the mother.

Chorionic villus sampling carries a 1 in 50 risk of causing a miscarriage and it is impossible to predict from the test whether the baby will be severely or mildly affected later in life.

CMT International UK's advice: Inevitably, views on the subject of testing will be coloured by an individual's own experience of CMT. Some couples cannot countenance having an affected child and opt for prenatal diagnosis and termination if the foetus is affected; others feel termination cannot be justified by the usually mild disability caused by CMT type 1a. We believe testing should **not be done** unless the couple is sure beforehand that they will terminate an affected pregnancy. There is nothing to be gained in knowing if the foetus has the duplicated gene for any other reason, and potentially much to be lost. Couples wishing to consider this option should seek referral to their nearest clinical genetics centre (see appendix 3).

The early testing of children for CMT

CMT type 1a can be detected by a blood test which can be carried out at any time after birth, even by taking a sample of blood from the umbilical cord. A fairly large sample is needed and some paediatricians advocate waiting until the child is at least eighteen months old.

Any family doctor can arrange a referral to the nearest clinical genetics centre for a blood test, though many centres are extremely reluctant to test a child with no symptoms. It can take between three to four months for the results to be known.

CMT International UK's advice: We believe early testing must be entirely the parents' decision and no-one else's. If after discussing all the implications with a suitable expert (such as a neurologist or a geneticist) you feel you can live with the results you must insist that your child is tested. Early testing combined with early physiotherapy or other treatments may have a positive long-term outcome.

How CMT is inherited

CMT International UK's advice: There is no reason why women with CMT cannot have children perfectly safely in the vast majority of cases. However, both prospective parents need to be fully aware of the genetic implications of their condition and should seek advice from a genetic counsellor before starting a family. Your family doctor can refer you.

There are three inheritance patterns for CMT, each of which is described below:

- Autosomal dominant inheritance (produces type 1a, type 1b, type 1c and all type 2 variants)
- Autosomal recessive inheritance (mainly type 4)
- X-linked inheritance.

A summary of the inheritance patterns in men and women

Men can inherit CMT in one of the following ways:

- if one parent has CMT (= autosomal dominant inheritance)
- if both parents are carriers (= autosomal recessive inheritance)
- if the mother is an X-linked carrier
- by a new mutation of the gene.

Women can inherit CMT in one of the following ways:

- if one parent has CMT (= autosomal dominant inheritance)
- if both parents are carriers of a recessive gene (= autosomal recessive inheritance)
- by a new mutation of the gene.

Autosomal dominant inheritance

The most common form of inheritance is *autosomal dominant* inheritance (figure 1). This means the affected person has one normal gene and one defective gene on the relevant pair of chromosomes. The condition affects men and women alike and each child of an affected parent has a 50 per cent chance of also being affected.[8]

Autosomal dominant is the inheritance pattern for CMT type 1a, type 1b, type 1c and all type 2 variants.

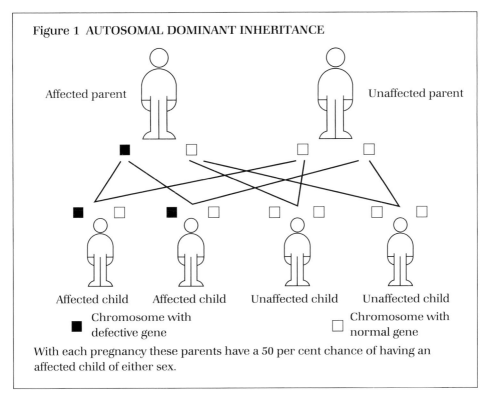

Figure 1 AUTOSOMAL DOMINANT INHERITANCE

Affected parent   Unaffected parent

Affected child   Affected child   Unaffected child   Unaffected child

■ Chromosome with defective gene   □ Chromosome with normal gene

With each pregnancy these parents have a 50 per cent chance of having an affected child of either sex.

Note that:

■ An unaffected child does not carry the defective gene and therefore cannot pass on CMT to his or her own children.

■ An affected child has the same 50 per cent chance of having an affected child as its parents.

---

8   It is possible for CMT type 1 to develop spontaneously in some individuals with normal parents. This *mutation* will be autosomal dominant and have a 50 per cent chance of being passed on to subsequent offspring (see also the next footnote).

Autosomal recessive inheritance

With type 4 the inheritance pattern is *autosomal recessive* inheritance (figure 2).[9] In such cases both parents are carriers; this means that although they do not display any symptoms themselves, each of their children – boys or girls – has a 25 per cent chance of inheriting a 'double dose' of the defective gene (ie, one from each parent) and therefore the condition will develop.

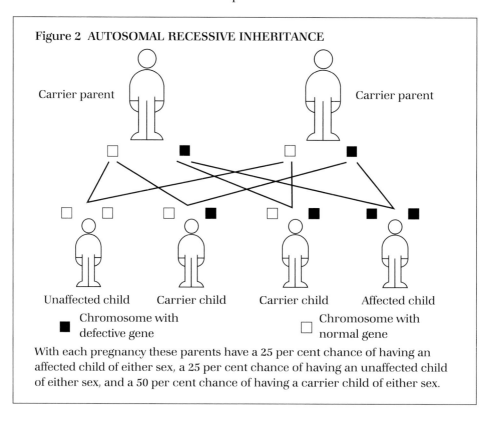

Figure 2 AUTOSOMAL RECESSIVE INHERITANCE

Carrier parent

Carrier parent

Unaffected child   Carrier child   Carrier child   Affected child

■ Chromosome with defective gene

□ Chromosome with normal gene

With each pregnancy these parents have a 25 per cent chance of having an affected child of either sex, a 25 per cent chance of having an unaffected child of either sex, and a 50 per cent chance of having a carrier child of either sex.

Many people with autosomal recessive CMT do not have affected relatives because the disorder only manifests itself in one set of brothers and sisters. Since only one in four of these brothers and sisters will be affected and most families are quite small, it is most likely that only one child will be affected.

---

9 It is worth noting that type 3 was long thought to be inherited in an autosomal recessive pattern. However, scientists now know that it is associated with a defect in the genes that are also involved in some forms of type 1 and that most cases result from a new mutation in the gene, which explains why neither parent is affected.

Note that:

■ An affected child can pass on CMT to his or her own children only if he or she is unfortunate enough to have a partner who is also a carrier of this type of CMT. In such cases the affected child has a 50 per cent chance of having an affected child of its own, but all the children will be carriers.

■ An unaffected child does not carry the defective gene and therefore cannot pass on CMT to his or her own children.

■ A carrier child (who is also unaffected) has a 50 per cent chance of having a child who is a carrier.

X-linked inheritance

In X-linked inheritance (figure 3) the defective gene is carried on one of the X chromosomes which determine the sex of the child. In this type of CMT the disease is passed on to the sons of a mother who is a carrier. Usually the mother will have no symptoms whatsoever or be only mildly affected. Each of the sons has a 50 per cent chance of having CMT, which is likely to be more severe than his mother's condition, and each of the daughters has a 50 per cent chance of being a carrier. Unaffected boys cannot pass on the condition to their sons.

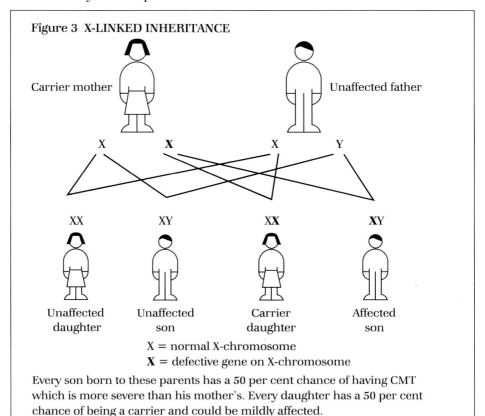

Figure 3 X-LINKED INHERITANCE

Carrier mother — Unaffected father

X   **X**   X   Y

XX — Unaffected daughter
XY — Unaffected son
X**X** — Carrier daughter
XY — Affected son

X = normal X-chromosome
X = defective gene on X-chromosome

Every son born to these parents has a 50 per cent chance of having CMT which is more severe than his mother's. Every daughter has a 50 per cent chance of being a carrier and could be mildly affected.

Note that:

- An affected father cannot pass on CMT to his sons but all his daughters will be carriers (see figure 4).

- A carrier mother has a 50 per cent chance of passing on CMT to her sons and a 50 per cent chance of her daughters being carriers.

- Any unaffected children cannot pass on CMT to their own children. There is no risk of any of them being carriers since they do not carry the defective gene.

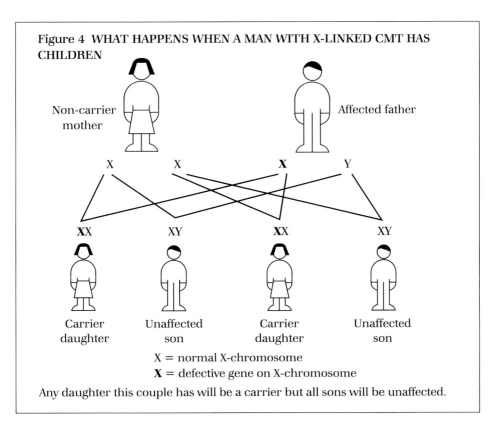

Figure 4 WHAT HAPPENS WHEN A MAN WITH X-LINKED CMT HAS CHILDREN

Non-carrier mother

Affected father

X   X   **X**   Y

XX   XY   **XX**   XY

Carrier daughter

Unaffected son

Carrier daughter

Unaffected son

X = normal X-chromosome
X = defective gene on X-chromosome

Any daughter this couple has will be a carrier but all sons will be unaffected.

Note: It is quite possible with all types of CMT for a person to have the defective gene within their *DNA* but to have no symptoms. This is why the condition may appear to 'skip' a generation in some families. However, there is still the same genetic risk to subsequent generations.

CMT and some other conditions

CMT and muscular dystrophy

CMT is **not** a form of muscular dystrophy. In muscular dystrophy the defect is within the muscles; in CMT it is in the nerves which supply the muscles.

CMT and multiple sclerosis

CMT type 1 and multiple sclerosis (MS) both involve demyelination of the nerves but they are two very different disorders. CMT affects the peripheral nerves whereas MS affects the central nervous system and the brain. CMT is a hereditary disorder. The exact cause of MS is unknown but evidence indicates that a virus or allergy might cause the body to turn against its own myelin.

CMT and Charcot's joint

CMT and Charcot's joint are two different disorders. Charcot's joint is a damaged and swollen joint.

CMT and distal spinal muscular atrophy

Distal spinal muscular atrophy (DSMA) is a disorder in which the nerve connections to the spinal cord are at fault rather than the myelin. Even so, CMT and DSMA are often confused because they produce very similar symptoms. The chief difference is that there is no sensory loss with DSMA.

CMT and hereditary neuropathy with liability to pressure palsies

Hereditary neuropathy with liability to pressure palsies (HNPP) and CMT are so similar genetically that misdiagnosis can occur. Like CMT type 1a, HNPP is a demyelinating form of neuropathy caused by an autosomal dominant gene. But while CMT type 1a results from having an extra copy of the myelin gene PMP22 on chromosome 17, HNPP results from a deletion of PMP22 which causes an irregular thickening of the myelin sheath.

HNPP causes episodes of numbness and weakness similar to an arm or a leg going to sleep (it is usually described as a painless disorder although some people do have pain which is probably a subjective sense of numbness). Episodes can last from several minutes to several months and may be triggered by stretching or pressure on the nerves. This may be the result of leaning on the elbows, kneeling, crossing the legs, cutting with scissors, knitting, or sleeping in the wrong position.

Most sufferers have normal strength and sensation unless they are experiencing an attack. Symptoms usually develop in the teenage years or early twenties and are typical of a more generalised hereditary motor and sensory neuropathy, which on occasion may be misdiagnosed as a form of CMT. Carpal tunnel syndrome[10] is frequently seen in people with HNPP.

Sufferers are usually advised to avoid activities that may cause the symptoms to develop, and crossing the legs and leaning on the elbows is discouraged. Ankle and foot orthoses can be used during periods of acute peroneal nerve palsy and for *foot drop* or balance problems.

As a hereditary neuropathy HNPP is progressive, though to what extent it will progress in any individual is unknown. There is no treatment or cure but it can now be diagnosed with a blood test.

---

10 A condition caused by the compression of the median nerve in the carpal tunnel and characterised especially by discomfort and disturbance of sensation in the hand.

CMT and stress

Stress is indicted as a factor in many illnesses from headaches to heart disease. Stress may aggravate an existing health problem or it may trigger an illness if a person is at risk for a particular condition. Situations that create stress are unique to each individual; personality, genes and experiences all influence how a person deals with stressors.

Generally, stress is what a person feels when the demands on their life exceed their ability to meet those demands. The stressor may be external, such as the death of a family member or close friend, or it may be an internal stressor such as an illness. Adults commonly list their top stressors as family, finances and work. Older people often find that social isolation is their biggest source of stress.

CMT can be a stressor, either at the time it is first diagnosed or later, when particular aspects of the condition begin to affect an individual.

Headaches, indigestion, sleeplessness and sweaty palms are common signs of stress, as are edginess, irritability and an inability to concentrate.

The stress response

Researchers do not completely understand how stress overlaps and interacts with physical illness. However, over the last twenty years a new field of study has emerged – psychoneuroimmunology – which focuses on how the central nervous system and the immune system[11] influence each other during stress.

Regardless of whether it is dealing with a frightful event or an ongoing tension in life, the body's physical response to any stressor is similar to its reaction to a physical threat: either it gears itself up to face the challenge ('fight') or it musters the strength to move out of harm's way ('flight').

A hormone called corticotropin releasing factor stimulates the pituitary gland in the brain to release adrenocorticotropic hormone. This signals the adrenal gland

---

11 The system that protects the body from foreign substances, cells and tissues by producing an immune response, including especially the thymus, spleen, lymph nodes, special deposits of lymphoid tissue (as in the gastrointestinal tract and bone marrow), lymphocytes (including the B-cells and T-cells) and immunoglobulins (including all known antibodies).

to release more hormones, including adrenaline (epinephrine) and cortisol. Epinephrine and cortisol prepare the body to respond to stress: the heart beats faster, breathing quickens and blood pressure rises. Blood carrying oxygen and nutrients is redirected to organs that need more energy to function under stress, such as the brain and muscles, while less blood goes to the stomach and skin.

At the same time potential energy sources – blood sugar (glucose) and fat – are released into the blood. Fibrin, a chemical that makes the blood clot more easily, is also released, perhaps to slow or stop bleeding in case of injury.

How stress and illness interact

Paradoxically, many of the physical reactions that help a person to fight or take flight can damage their health in the long run:

- **The immune system** – Cortisol produced during the stress response may suppress the immune system and thus increase the body's susceptibility to infectious diseases. Studies suggest that bacterial infections such as tuberculosis and group A streptococcal disease increase during stress. Stress may also make a person prone to upper respiratory viral infections such as colds and flu.

- **Cardiovascular disease** – Under acute stress the heart beats quickly making people more susceptible to angina and heart rhythm irregularities. If someone is a 'hot reactor' acute stress may add to their risk of having a heart attack (as a response to daily stress hot reactors exhibit extreme increases in heart rate and blood pressure which may gradually result in injury to the coronary arteries and the heart). Increased blood clotting as a result of the stress response can increase the risk of heart attack or stroke. Research suggests stress can also lead to chronic high blood pressure in people with no family history of the condition.

The relationship between stress and other illnesses is not so clear cut. But stress may worsen symptoms if a person is prone to these conditions:

- **Asthma** – A stressful situation can make the airways over-reactive thus precipitating an attack.

- **Gastrointestinal problems** – Stress can make the symptoms worse in people who have a gastrointestinal disorder such as an ulcer or irritable bowel syndrome.

Some commonly used techniques for dealing with stress can be found on page 55.

CMT and anaesthesia

People with CMT or other neuromuscular disorders[12] must take great care if they are to have a general or local anaesthetic. Even someone with very mild symptoms – or no symptoms at all – or someone who has a family history of a disorder **must** let the anaesthetist know well in advance so that the appropriate tests can be carried out and proper after-care can be arranged. **It is for this reason that people with CMT and other neuromuscular disorders may not be suitable for treatment as day cases.**

The main areas of concern are how the anaesthetic gases or chemicals will affect the nerves and muscle tissue, and especially how they will affect the heart. A skeletal deformity such as scoliosis can also affect the way a person responds to anaesthesia.

Doctors may sometimes measure the strength of a person's muscles by assessing the amount of physical activity they can perform and by taking a blood sample to measure the levels of creatine kinase, a muscle enzyme.

Anaesthetics and breathing

Any anaesthetic agent which affects the muscles will affect the lungs. The muscles used for swallowing can also be affected. Strong analgesic or sedative agents will affect these muscles indirectly while muscle relaxants will have a direct effect. As breathing may already be difficult for a person with a neuromuscular disorder, these drugs should be used with caution, and the monitoring of breathing after an operation is essential. In fact, good post-operative care is so important for people with neuromuscular disorders that they are best cared for in a high dependency unit or an intensive care unit immediately after an operation.

Muscle relaxants

Muscle relaxant drugs tend to have a more profound and prolonged effect on someone with a neuromuscular disorder compared with other patients and should only be used if absolutely necessary.

12 A list of neuromuscular disorders is on page 34.

One type of muscle relaxant, suxamethonium, should usually be avoided. Suxamethonium causes the release of potassium ions from the muscle tissue into the blood. In normal patients this is usually of little practical significance but in patients with a neuromuscular disorder the muscle may be 'leaking' potassium ions into the blood already and a further increase may cause abnormal heart rhythms. A pre-operative blood test to check the level of potassium ions in the blood is therefore very important.[13]

Local anaesthetics

A local anaesthetic works by preventing the normal electrical activity in the nerves around which the anaesthetic agent is placed. For minor procedures such as stitching a cut a local anaesthetic is probably the best choice for someone with a neuromuscular disorder because there are few, if any, side-effects. However, for major local anaesthetic procedures – spinal or epidural, for example – careful assessment of the patient is needed and the type of disorder must be considered long before the operation.

Changes in body temperature and pre-operative 'starvation'

A person with a neuromuscular disorder will not easily tolerate changes in body temperature or the starvation often associated with anaesthesia so steps need to be taken to minimise these problems by keeping the patient warm and well hydrated.

CMT International UK's advice: It is absolutely essential that the anaesthetist is aware of your condition well in advance of the operation even if your CMT symptoms are minor or you have no symptoms at all. (Occasionally a neuromuscular disorder has come to light only because of an unexpected problem with anaesthesia, particularly in young children.) The anaesthetist should also be warned if there is an inherited neuromuscular disorder in your family. Consider wearing a Medic Alert bracelet in case you are in an accident, and if you are going to have an operation you could show the anaesthetist this book beforehand.

---

13 A list of other drugs which may affect or exacerbate CMT is on page 35.

Neuromuscular disorders

Neuromuscular disorders include all the muscular dystrophies plus:

- Hereditary and idiopathic peripheral neuropathy (Charcot-Marie-Tooth disease)

- Myotonic disorders

- Congenital myopathies, including mini-core, central-core and multi-core disease plus nemaline and myotubular myopathies

- Mitochondrial myopathies

- Lipid storage myopathies

- Inherited metabolic myopathies, including glycogen storage disease

- Familial periodic paralysis

- Inflammatory myopathies, including infective myositis

- Autoimmune myositides, including polymyositis and dermatomyositis

- Spinal muscular atrophies

- Inflammatory, autoimmune and toxic neuropathies, including Guillain Barre syndrome and CIDP

- Disorders of the neuromuscular junction, including myasthenia gravis

Drugs which may affect or exacerbate CMT

Before taking any medication be sure to discuss it fully with your doctor or pharmacist for possible side effects. Ask them to look for the words 'could cause peripheral neuropathy' in the drug description. In almost all the conditions in which these drugs are used an alternative is available.

These drugs are toxic to the peripheral nervous system and may be harmful to a person with CMT:

Drugs used in the treatment of cancer

- Doxorubicin/Adriamycin
- Cisplatinum
- Misomidazole (can be used with caution)
- Suramin
- Taxol
- Vincristine

Drugs used in the treatment of tuberculosis

- Ethionamide
- Isoniazid (INH)

Drugs used in the treatment of heart conditions

- Cordarone-X – for irregular heartbeat
- Hydralazine (Apresoline) – for high blood pressure
- Perhexiline (Pexid) – for angina

Anaesthetics

- Nitrous oxide/Entonox
- Succinylcholine (suxamenthonium, Anectine)

Other drugs

- Chloramphenicol – an antibiotic
- Dapsone – for chronic and certain rare skin diseases
- Phenytoin (Epanutin) – for seizures and pain
- Disulfiram (Antabuse) – for alcoholics

- Flagyl (Metronidazol) – for trichomonas infection[14]
- Glutethimide (Doriden) – a sleeping pill
- Lithium – for manic depressive illness or headaches (use with caution)
- Nitrofurantoin (Furadantin, Macrobid, Macrodantin) – for urinary tract infection
- Penicillamine – for rheumatoid arthritis

Vitamins

Megadoses of vitamins A, B6 (Pyridoxine) and D can be harmful. A megadose is defined as ten times the recommended daily allowance.

Other substances

- Alcohol
- Tobacco

> **CMT International UK's advice:** It is important to remember that these are possible risks rather than proven risks. We believe it would be a tragedy if someone were to be denied effective treatment because of anxieties about unproven risks.

---

14 Can be found in combination with other drugs for vaginal yeast infections. Also used topically for acne and orally as an antibiotic by some dentists and doctors.

CMT and complementary medicine

The human body is a complex self-healing organism which works constantly to fight infection, heal wounds and remove toxins from the body. Its natural tendency is towards balanced health and harmony. Over the past decade there has been a great deal of interest in harnessing and working with these natural healing processes, or 'life energies', as an alternative to traditional medical practice. This activity is known as complementary medicine.

At present anyone in the UK can set themselves up as a practitioner of a wide variety of complementary therapies. Standardisation and validation of training and quality standards is urgently needed and is being addressed at a national level.

If you are interested in finding out more about complementary medicine as a possible treatment for CMT you should consult the British Register of Complementary Practitioners or the Institute for Complementary Therapists for a list of practitioners or courses in your area. The addresses of both organisations can be found in appendix 2.

Some useful books on the subject are: *The Greening Of Medicine* (Gollancz) and *Holistic Living* (Dent), both by Patrick Pietroni, and *The Handbook Of Complementary Medicine* by Stephen Fulder (Coronet).

CMT International UK's advice: If you have a health problem it is advisable to always consult your family doctor first and discuss the various options that may be open to you. If you subsequently seek help from a practitioner of complementary medicine it is very important to check their credentials.

Glossary of scientific and medical terms

1 Terms used in this book

Amino acids – The chemical building blocks of proteins. Twenty different amino acids are found in the proteins in the human body. The sequence of amino acids in a protein is determined by the genetic code.

Autosomal – All the chromosomes other than the sex chromosomes are known as autosomes. Human beings have 22 pairs of autosomes. Autosomal inheritance means that a defective gene can affect either sex.

Axon – The long projection of a neurone.

Biopsy – The surgical removal of a small amount of nerve or muscle tissue for examination in the laboratory.

Carrier – A healthy individual who has one copy of a gene associated with a recessive genetic disease and one normal copy of the gene. The disease will not manifest itself in that person because the normal gene is sufficient for normal functioning, but the defective copy may be transmitted to subsequent generations.

Cell – The smallest unit of a living organism that can survive independently and reproduce itself. It has been estimated that the adult body consists of 50 billion cells. Inside the cell is a structure called the nucleus which contains all the DNA of the organism.

Chorionic villus sampling – A prenatal screening procedure in which the cells of the chorion, a membrane surrounding the embryo, are withdrawn for genetic analysis. The chorionic villi are situated on the wall of the uterus (womb) and form the early placenta (afterbirth). They have the same genetic make-up as the unborn baby and can be tested to detect certain abnormalities.

Chromosomes – Sausage-shaped bundles in the cell nucleus made of a very long strand of the chemical DNA coiled upon itself many times. Human beings have 22 pairs of autosomal chromosomes and one pair of sex chromosomes. Fertilisation of a 23-chromosome egg by a 23-chromosome sperm produces a new 46-chromosome cell which grows into a new individual. One half of each chromosome pair is inherited from each parent.

DNA – Deoxyribonucleic acid, the chemical of which genes are made. DNA contains coded information arranged in a linear sequence. The chromosomes in each cell contain about two metres of DNA.

Dominant – A dominant gene exercises the same outward effect when inherited from only one parent as when inherited from both. Alterations in genes (mutations) which lead to an abnormal functioning of the corresponding protein can cause inherited disorders.

Foot drop – A condition in which the ankle cannot be flexed upward towards the knee.

Gene – The basic physical and functional unit of heredity that is transmitted from one generation to the next. Composed of sequences of bases in DNA. Human beings are estimated to have between 50,000–100,000 genes. Genes are inherited in pairs, one from each parent.

Genetics – That part of biology dealing with the constancy of inheritance and its variation. The study of the replication, transmission and expression of hereditary information.

Genetic counsellor – A specialist who provides information and support to people who have genetic conditions in their families or who are concerned about the possibility of genetically transmitted conditions in the future.

Genetic disorders – Conditions resulting from defects in the genetic make-up of an individual, either in single genes or whole chromosomes, parts of which may be lost, duplicated or transposed in the strand of DNA.

Mutation – A molecular event in which the DNA is altered with genetic consequences.

Myelin – A substance which covers the axon like the insulation around a wire and helps it to transmit messages quickly over long distances in the body. Demyelinating diseases damage this covering but spare the actual nerve fibre.

Orthoses – Devices or aids to prevent, correct or control physical deformities.

Prenatal – Before birth.

Protein – A large molecule composed of one or more chains of amino acids. Proteins are essential to the structure and functioning of cells and play a part in all the biological functions of an organism.

Recessive – A form of inheritance in which a genetic defect causes little or no outward effect unless it is present in both of a pair of genes (and has therefore been inherited from both parents). If a person inherits one defective gene and one normal gene, he or she will not be affected but will be a carrier. If two carriers of the same defective gene have children there is a 25 per cent chance in each pregnancy that the child will inherit two copies of the defective gene and will therefore be affected.

Sex chromosomes – The X and Y chromosomes determine the sex of an individual. Females have two X chromosomes; males have an X and a Y chromosome. Females are therefore described as XX and males as XY.

2 Other terms commonly encountered in genetic counselling

Allele – One of several possible forms of a gene. There might be alleles relating to either blue eyes or brown eyes, for example. Alleles are inherited separately from each parent.

Amniocentesis – Removal of a sample of amniotic fluid for prenatal testing. Cells from the unborn child can be extracted from the fluid which surrounds it in the womb and tested for abnormalities. Usually taken after 16 weeks.

Atrophy – The thinning or wasting away of muscle tissue after prolonged disuse. Can occur when CMT nerves no longer provide the muscles with the impulses to move.

Cardiac – To do with the heart.

Carrier testing – A test to find out if a person who does not show symptoms of a condition nevertheless carries a defective gene which could be passed on to his or her children.

Congenital disorder – A condition that is present at birth.

Contractures – A shortening of the muscles or tendons which prevents the associated joints from moving freely.

Cytogenetics – The study of the number and structure of the chromosomes.

Deletion – The loss of genetic material from a chromosome or gene.

Double helix – The usual configuration of DNA consisting of two complementary strands, each made up of long repeating strands, running side by side in a helical formation and joined together by the bases.

Electromyography – A diagnostic test for many types of neuromuscular disorders involving the insertion of a small needle into several muscles to obtain information about the severity and cause of the weakness. It is usually combined with nerve conduction studies which measure the integrity of various motor and sensory nerves.

Foetal therapy – The treatment of the foetus before birth, either directly or indirectly through the administration of drugs to the mother.

Gamete – A reproductive cell (sperm or ova in mammals).

Gene enhancement – The insertion of additional genetic material into an otherwise normal genome to enhance a trait that is perceived as desirable.

Gene therapy – The replacement or repair of defective genes in living cells.

Genetic code – The sequence of nucleotides that determines the sequence of amino acids in the creation of a protein.

Genetic engineering – The technique of altering the genetic make-up of cells or individual organisms by deliberately inserting, removing or altering genes.

Genetic markers – Harmless variations in the DNA which lie close to the site of a disrupted gene and which may be used for tracking a condition through a family.

Genetic screening – The process of systematically scanning individual genotypes for possible hereditary defects or abnormalities.

Genome – The entire genetic endowment of an organism or a species, usually expressed as the total number of base pairs. The human genome, for example, is approximately three billion base pairs in length.

Genotype – The genetic make-up underlying a specific trait or constellation of traits.

Heredity – The transmission of base pairs from parents to their children.

Heterozygous – Means the copies of each gene inherited from each parent are different.

Homozygous – Means the copies of each gene inherited from each parent are identical.

In vitro fertilisation (IVF) – Fertilisation outside the body. Occurs literally 'in the glass', as in a test tube.

Immune response – The response by the body to 'foreign' material such as a transplanted organ or an infection.

Linkage studies – Tests carried out on various family members to establish which piece of genetic code is causing a particular condition in that family.

Muscle fibre – The basic unit of muscle tissue which is formed by the fusion of groups of muscle cells.

Mutagen – An agent that increases the incidence of genetic mutation. Examples include radiation and certain kinds of chemicals.

Nucleus – The structure in the centre of each cell which contains the chromosomes and their genetic material.

Phenotype – The detectable physical characteristics associated with a particular genotype.

Polygenic trait – A trait whose transmission involves more than one gene.

Preclinical diagnosis – Diagnosis of a genetic disorder before there are any symptoms.

Prognosis – The predicted course and outcome of a disorder.

Somatic cell – Any cell in the body other than germ cells.

Trait – A character difference in an organism for which a gene is responsible.

Ultrasound – A technique using reflected high frequency sound waves to produce images of muscle structure, internal organs and babies in the womb.

Zygote – A fertilised egg.

Part 2
Living with CMT

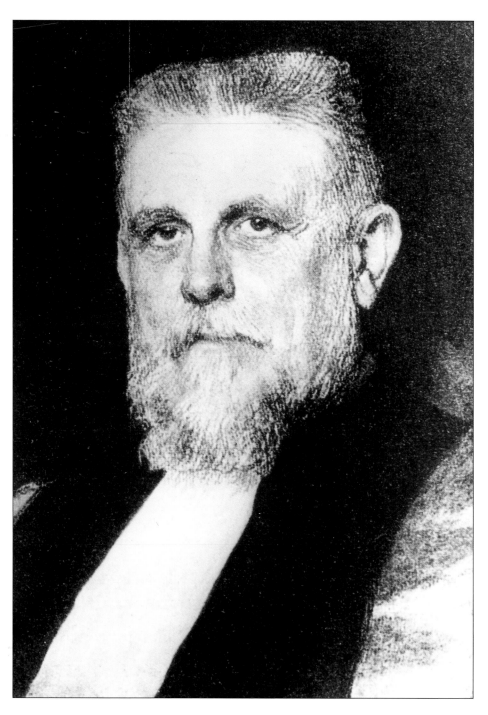

Plate II Pierre Marie

The impact of CMT on each stage of life

CMT is a lifelong condition which impacts on people in different ways throughout their lives. To appreciate how CMT might affect a person at each stage of life it is useful to consider the theories of the psychologist Erik Erikson, who first popularised the notion of life as a series of 'tasks to be accomplished' in order to pass on successfully to the next stage.

Erikson's five stages of life – infancy, the toddler stage, childhood, puberty and young adulthood – define the periods which everyone passes through and delineate the times when people may be more vulnerable to certain aspects of CMT.

Stage 1 Infancy

CMT is not usually obvious during infancy. However, if it is known to run in the family, or if the child has had a DNA test for the types of CMT which can be tested for, a close observer might notice early signs.

The real impact of CMT at this stage is from parental feelings of passing on a trait which is less than desirable. If parents have not come to terms with their own CMT and feel guilty or depressed, interaction with their infant may be affected.

First-born children, especially those who have no siblings or are born late in life, tend to be scrutinised by their parents, with all their deficiencies and accomplishments magnified and ruminated upon.

Erikson's life-task at this stage is for the infant to develop trust in its parents and in the world around it – something that happens when unconditional love is given and received.

> **CMT International UK's advice:** What can a parent do at this stage? Ignore the possibility of CMT and enjoy your baby!

Stage 2 The toddler stage

During this stage children accomplish their 'motor milestones': they learn to walk, to control their bladders and bowels, and to handle simple utensils and toys. Some children begin to show signs of CMT at this stage, being slower to walk or walking clumsily.

Erikson's life-task at this stage is to overcome shame and doubt and develop a sense of autonomy or control over the body. It is the parent who gives the child a sense of autonomy by praising his or her efforts and successes; this is the beginning of self-esteem. If the parent is ashamed of the child's clumsiness or doubts its abilities, the child will sense this.

CMT International UK's advice: If your toddler's CMT is severe (though this would be unusual) then therapy from a physiotherapist or occupational therapist specialising in paediatrics might prove helpful in improving strength and motor patterns. Each child develops at its own pace, in its own way – and each child needs parents who can accept and encourage it.

Stage 3 Childhood

During early and late childhood children are busy learning about themselves and the world around them. Their ability to think and reason changes as they grow. During early childhood (approximately 3–6 years of age) their thought processes are concrete: they think in terms of the present and what they can actually see. As they mature their mental capacity allows them to think more abstractly. By late childhood (ages 7–12) they can imagine the future, think of different possibilities and appreciate logical consequences.

Children might begin to be aware of their CMT during this phase of their growth. Erikson's life-tasks at this stage are learning initiative and industry. If children become afraid to take chances because of repeated physical failure or teasing by their peers they may experience what Erikson called 'guilt' or 'inferiority'. If their sense of discovery, adventure and willingness to try something new is thwarted by feelings of failure they may enter adolescence with an inferiority complex and feel guilty for 'not trying harder'.

As they leave the childhood stages children should feel competent about their ability to cope with life and that they are keeping up with their peers within their capacity.

CMT International UK's advice: During the childhood stages parents should help their children to discover their best selves by being open and truthful with them, encouraging them to do well in all their life-tasks, providing extra praise for what they do best, and maintaining perspective and a sense of humour.

Stage 4 Puberty

Adolescence is the stage that most adults, with or without CMT, report as being the most difficult. Children are at their most vulnerable and self-conscious at this stage, scrutinising every thought and action, wanting to appear like everyone else (to fit in) but at the same time wanting to be admired for being their own unique selves.

Erikson's life-task in this phase is to form an identity. Children need to maintain a positive self-image, to feel confident in their ability to interact and make their way in the world. Rebellion is a way of testing limits and many adolescents discover their limits by engaging in unsafe, unrealistic or unacceptable behaviour. A child who may have acknowledged his or her CMT in the past might seem to deny it at this stage in their choice of physical activity or career. Adolescents tend to be risk-takers who feel nothing can stand in their way. This powerful feeling does not correlate with having a potentially limiting neurological condition.

CMT International UK's advice: The lines of communication, sense of humour and perspective that were established during childhood are very important during adolescence. So is an open mind. But the truth of the matter is that an identity cannot always be forged under the umbrella of parental guidance.

Stage 5 Young adulthood

At some point in their early to mid-twenties adolescents turn into young adults and become self-sufficient. Although environmental factors and family values will influence lifestyle, most young adults will live away from home and be gainfully employed. Many will have started their own families.

The issues that emerge during this phase are all about careers and partners. Erikson's life-task is 'intimacy vs isolation'. To become a functioning partner in an intimate relationship requires a positive sense of self. This stage is problematical for all young adults, not just for those with CMT. And choosing a career can be just as tricky as choosing a mate, especially when weighing and balancing the possible effects of a progressive neuropathy.

At some point in a person's adult years the biological aspects of CMT will come to the fore: foot drop, decreasing stamina, hand weakness, poor balance. Any combination of these symptoms may necessitate changing or, in extreme cases, giving up a career.

CMT International UK's advice: By this stage young adults will be going their own way. Parents should listen to their plans, validate their feelings and support them as much as they are able. But they should also live their own lives as fully as possible and hope that their example will be appreciated by their children.

Coming to terms with CMT

Any chronic disabling condition can affect the way people feel and think about themselves. People with CMT often suffer from low self-esteem, and relationships at work and within the family may be affected.[15]

As a person learns to live with CMT the possibility of losing the ability to play tennis, use a computer, do up zips and buttons, or turn the pages of a newspaper, can affect their perception of self over and over again.

> **CMT International UK's advice:** A grieving period can occur at every loss. Talking about these reactions with an understanding person is far better than resorting to mood-altering drugs. A spouse, relative, counsellor or other professional person who understands CMT and can deal with the grieving process for a lost body function is one of the most valuable allies a person with CMT can have.

When a child is diagnosed

Many parents have said that the diagnosis of CMT was just the beginning of a wide range of emotions that they would eventually experience. These emotions do not follow any set pattern or last a set amount of time. They are, however, honest reactions and valid responses to the family's circumstances, and might include:

- **Denial and disbelief** – Some parents say they had a feeling long before the diagnosis was made that something was wrong. In many cases, with a hereditary disorder, they are waiting for what they most fear – the same diagnosis that plagued their own youth – but they deny those feelings until their fears are confirmed. This is a healthy reaction; it gives a person time to accept, adjust, and make plans. It can also protect a parent from too much pain too soon.

---

15 The Association to Aid the Sexual and Personal Relationships of People with a Disability (SPOD) operates a telephone counselling line and produces advisory leaflets, information sheets and resource lists for anyone who is experiencing sexual or relationship difficulties. The number is in appendix 2.

■ **Sadness and depression** – Many parents say they experienced depression when their child was diagnosed with CMT. If the child is the first family member to be diagnosed, the depression is likely to be a direct result of the ignorance of how serious the condition might become. Often, depression or depressed feelings may occur unexpectedly, without the person knowing why. Sadness may be associated with the dreams and expectations the parents had for their child's life and their own: seeing other children doing something that your child cannot do or cannot do without pain and difficulty can trigger long-buried feelings of sadness.

■ **Anger and hostility** – It is not uncommon for parents to direct their anger towards the doctor who diagnosed their child, or towards each other, or towards the child. Often they will hear themselves saying, 'It's not fair' or 'Life isn't fair'. It is perfectly normal to feel anger at the unjustness of having a disability.

■ **Fear** – Fear is a common reaction to the unknown. When parents are told their child will not be 'typical' they feel apprehensive. When that general fear is coupled with uncertainty about what the future may hold for someone with CMT, because of its variable nature, parents are often doubly fearful. It is normal to feel anxious about an uncertain future, to feel inadequate as a parent, and to become over protective in order to help you deal with the situation.

CMT International UK's advice: The important thing to remember is that all parents experience different emotions about their child's diagnosis and development. It is healthy, normal and very common to feel angry, afraid, guilty and sad. Once a parent can identify and acknowledge these feelings, he or she can begin to use some of the strategies for coping (see opposite).

Strategies for coping

Cognitive coping

- Read everything you can find on your child's disability
- Talk to the parents of a child with a similar diagnosis
- Subscribe to newsletters on CMT (see appendix 1)
- Attend workshops and conferences on CMT

Physical coping

- Cry, laugh, have a sense of humour
- Keep a journal. Write down your emotions and the coping mechanism that worked for you
- Exercise
- Eat well
- Rest sufficiently
- Take long walks
- Keep a normal routine

Psychological coping

- Join a support group or start one (see appendix 1)
- Take up your child's cause by raising the awareness of others
- Take one day at a time
- Replace negative thoughts with positive ones
- Mentally list all the wonderful things your child can do
- Realise you are not alone
- Get counselling if you need it
- Find a parent who has been in a similar situation

Spiritual coping

- Talk to your family priest, minister, or rabbi

Tips for staying healthy

Health and self-responsibility

Most people with CMT have basically healthy bodies, but like anyone else they have a responsibility to look after themselves. By taking a few simple precautions many general health problems can be avoided:

- Circulation in limbs that are not working at full capacity can be a problem, so feet and hands should be kept warm. Chilblains are an unnecessary problem and should be avoided at all costs.

- Do not risk pressure sores. People who spend a lot of time in a wheelchair should make sure they have a decent pressure-relieving cushion (available through an occupational therapist) and ensure they stretch out on a bed from time to time.

- People with CMT should take extra care to avoid falling because fractures take longer to heal and the resulting inactivity may cause the CMT to worsen. Falls can be prevented by wearing proper shoes (with orthoses, if necessary – see page 65) and by taking care on uneven ground.

General exercise

It is important for people with CMT to maintain what movement, muscles and strength they may have, and to stay flexible for as long as possible. However, any exercise that causes prolonged fatigue can be detrimental.

Movements should be made as easy as possible to prevent overuse of the affected muscle groups. In this way, flexibility will be preserved and unwanted secondary complications can be minimised or avoided. Anyone starting out on an exercise regime should build up a routine gradually, with extreme caution, and preferably under the supervision of a trained instructor. Wherever possible, a physiotherapist who understands the disease process of CMT should devise a personalised exercise programme.

Swimming is an excellent form of exercise since it does not put any undue stress on the joints. Many leisure centres have clubs for disabled swimmers.

CMT International UK's advice: Choose exercises that you can do at your own pace without being pressured into pushing yourself. Bear in mind that overuse of any particular set of muscles will have a detrimental effect on those muscles. If you are considering body-building be aware that it is impossible to build up muscle bulk on muscles that have already atrophied through CMT.

Nutrition

People with CMT should try to eat a healthy diet with a low calorie content. Obesity resulting from overeating or inactivity should be avoided at all costs because:

■ it decreases the availability of oxygen to the tissues. Oxygen is necessary for the proper functioning of every cell in the body.

■ it compromises physical performance. Physical activity becomes more difficult, which is the last thing a person with CMT needs.

■ it raises the 'energy cost' of activity. An obese person requires more energy to perform a task than a lean person.

■ it increases the demands on the heart and lungs.

■ it increases the stress on the joints. CMT joints are already stressed from the disorder and extra weight on muscles, ligaments, tendons and joints can be a real source of pain.

Alcohol may be drunk **in moderation**. A large amount can irritate the already damaged nerves.

CMT International UK's advice: Always consult your family doctor before launching into a new diet. Approach drastic diets with extreme caution, since they may weaken you.

Care of the feet

People with CMT often find it difficult to obtain well fitting shoes because of their arched feet. It is important to always wear shoes with good support, and arch supports or other devices within the shoes may be needed. People with weak leg muscles may find plastic splints useful in reducing the tendency of the foot to drop.

Ideally, children and teenagers with CMT should be seen annually by a paediatrician or neurologist to help ensure that foot problems do not develop. Surgery may be helpful for very highly arched feet, either to reduce the arch and the curling of the toes which often goes with it, or to fuse together some of the bones (see page 64).

The feet should also be checked regularly by a chiropodist. If the sensory nerves are not working properly an in-growing toenail or an ulcer may not be felt. These can be dealt with easily if caught in time but can cause problems if left too long.

People who have a lot of numbness in their feet should take great care to wash and dry them carefully and inspect the skin regularly. Shoes should be shaken out to remove small stones and the insides felt for irregularities which could damage the skin.

CMT International UK's advice: If the neurologist you see is not familiar with the condition we may be able to advise you on finding one who is, but this may involve travelling some distance to see them.

Breathing problems

In very rare cases CMT can affect the muscles that control breathing. This can manifest itself in the form of severe headaches, particularly in the morning. This happens because the body's breathing pattern changes at night to give deeper, slower breaths. If the lungs are not functioning properly this pattern is disrupted, resulting in carbon dioxide being retained in the body, hence the headaches.

It is important to have this problem checked thoroughly by a specialist. A sleep study in hospital can confirm what the problem is, and it can usually be cured either by the use of a supportive respirator or drugs which alter the sleep pattern.

Dealing with stress

■ **Change the factors you can** – Few people are in a position to walk away from a stressful job or home environment but they can learn to develop new responses to defuse anger or conflict. They can also learn to better manage their time by using a variety of techniques from delegating household responsibilities to just saying 'No'.

■ **Exercise regularly** – The natural decrease in adrenaline after exercise may counteract the stress response. People who are physically fit handle stress better. (For more about the types of exercise that are most suitable for people with CMT see above. For more about the body's response to stress see page 30.)

■ **Relax** – Use techniques such as guided imagery, meditation, muscle relaxation and relaxed breathing to help you to relax. The goal is to lower the heart rate and blood pressure while reducing muscle tension.

■ **Find a friend** – Social support can help to reduce stress and prolong life.

■ **Recognise when you need help** – If stress is keeping you from work or other activities talk to your doctor or a specialist in behavioural medicine. Behavioural therapy is one approach that can help you gain control over your symptoms.

CMT International UK's advice: This quick exercise will help you to relax your breathing. It can have an immediate calming effect when you are faced with a stressful situation. (1) To a count of four, inhale slowly. Imagine the inhaled warm air flowing to all parts of your body. (2) Pause. (3) Slowly exhale, again counting to four. Imagine the tension flowing out. (4) Pause, then begin again. Repeat several times.

Hints on conserving energy

People with progressive CMT may find they need to modify many areas of their life in order to cope with the fatigue that goes with their condition. By conserving energy in less important areas it is possible for them to continue with the activities that they enjoy.

Here are a few ideas which may be helpful:

DO rest before you become aware of fatigue. Before starting an activity decide how long you will work and when you will take rest breaks. For stressful projects set a timer and break the activity into segments of thirty minutes' work and fifteen minutes' rest. Lie down during your rest break.

DO NOT be over ambitious on days when you feel good or you may be fatigued for several days afterwards. Alternate light and heavy chores throughout the week. Do not do anything heavy if you are planning an evening activity.

DO sit whenever possible: for showering, dressing, grooming, preparing meals, etc. Sitting uses 25 per cent less energy than standing. When you sit make sure that your work surface is about an inch below elbow level. A drafting chair on casters with a pneumatic seat lift is ideal.

DO NOT put away items that you use frequently. For example, leave pans to dry on top of the cooker after washing up. Let dishes dry in a rack and then use them in setting the table for the next meal.

DO rearrange your home to minimise trips. Install floor-to-ceiling shelving over the toilet tank in the bathroom for storing towels and washcloths. Store sheets and pillowcases in the bedrooms where they are used. In the kitchen store frequently used items at a height between your hips and your lips. Use stacking storage bins on wheels and wire shelf units that hook over cupboard doors. Sliding racks, bins, baskets and shelf trays can make base cabinets for food staples and cleaning supplies.

DO NOT buy deep-pile carpets with thick padding or rugs that can slip. Wheelchair users find plush carpeting difficult to manoeuvre on and people with mobility problems may have difficulty maintaining their balance.

DO   duplicate household supplies in different areas. For example, store cleansers and sponges under each sink and keep a broom and a dust pan in several locations.

DO   use mechanical help such as a kitchen utility trolley or lightweight luggage cart for moving things around the home. Use a trolley to carry laundry and cleaning items or to transport articles between the car, house and office, and to move heavy articles from room to room.

Pain and pain control

The sources of pain

Most people with CMT experience pain. It is either sharp, sudden and short-lived or gnawing, long-lasting chronic pain. It can be pain associated with dysfunctional nerves, where the muscles are called upon to do many times their original job because other muscles have atrophied, or pain from trying to work a normal day or from too much work or play.

Most pain is not caused by the CMT-affected nerves themselves but by something that has atrophied or weakened because of the malfunctioning CMT nervous system. For example, the nerves that serve the muscles in the feet do not function correctly because they are affected by CMT, which means that the muscles in the feet are weakened, which means that extra strain is put on the ligaments and joints. The ligaments weaken because the foot muscles are not playing their part and the joints weaken because the ligaments are not playing their part. The messages to the muscles are leaving the brain correctly but are not reaching the muscles properly. The end result is misshapen and painful feet.

CMT International UK's advice: Pain can have a psychological as well as a physical source. It can be caused by worry, stress, fear, depression, grief, anger. Before turning to a doctor for pain relief it is important to first make sure that you have done everything in your power to help your body and mind stay as healthy and pain free as possible. If you have not accepted the fact that you have CMT you could be fighting a losing battle.

Dealing with pain

It is much more difficult to relieve pain after it has become established so people with CMT should learn to recognise the signs and do something about it before it takes hold.

Doctors are becoming more and more experienced in pain control and have a huge arsenal of drugs at their command. Addiction is rarely a concern when pain control drugs are used correctly. However, it takes doctors who know CMT and doctors who know drugs to combine their knowledge to help the person with CMT to control their pain.

Pain clinics have the means to diagnose various kinds of pain and to measure its severity, and they can teach a person to control their pain as much as possible. They generally use a multi-disciplinary approach which may include drugs, alternative therapies like TENS machines (which block nerve impulses), acupuncture, chiropractics, physiotherapy, private counselling and group therapy, depending on the type of pain and what is causing it.

As a final resort CMT pain can be relieved by surgery. If nerves become trapped and chronically painful a nerve block can sometimes be very effective. Orthopaedic surgery can also help – a triple arthrodesis, for example, can produce a balanced foot and thereby relieve the stresses and strains on other parts of the body (see page 66).

> **CMT International UK's advice:** Too many doctors try to deny a person with CMT their pain or give up after two or three attempts to control it. If a doctor denies your pain with CMT, find another one or ask to be referred to a pain clinic.

Preventing secondary complications

CMT is a complex disorder since the type of muscle weakness and sensory loss and the degree of disability it produces varies so considerably between individuals. In this respect the type of CMT a person has does not make a great deal of difference since no type indicates a specific pattern of muscle weakness. All people with CMT show different problems in relation to the severity and distribution of the muscles that are affected.

All people with CMT should have their movements analysed by a physiotherapist. A physiotherapist cannot stop the disease progressing, but because they understand movement they can spot potential problems which may arise as a result of an individual's particular weakness and thus help to prevent secondary complications.

In cases where there is a major muscle imbalance and the foot is being constantly pulled inwards it may be necessary to consider corrective surgery. Surgery was very prevalent in the past as a way of 'managing' the CMT foot. These days the use of splints before shortening develops means that surgery can often be avoided. (For more about orthopaedic surgery see page 64.)

Foot impairment and its influence on walking

The majority of people with CMT experience weakness and sensory loss in the feet and hands. In most cases the first symptoms are seen in the feet: high arches and clawing of the toes, both of which are caused by muscle imbalance.

The muscles which lift the foot upwards and outwards are usually more affected than those which push the foot downwards and inwards. The muscle on the outside of the calf which pulls the foot upwards and outwards is very important for balance. It passes underneath the foot and attaches to the base of the big toe. Its action in standing is to keep the foot firmly on the ground. Weakness in this muscle will cause instability at the ankle joint and the foot will tend to turn inwards. It is for this reason that many people with CMT often sprain their ankles.

As the CMT progresses and the feet become weaker it becomes more difficult to lift the toes clear of the ground when taking a step forwards. To compensate for this the legs are lifted higher by bending more at the hips and knees. The danger of this way of walking is that the calf muscle and the Achilles tendon will shorten and affect the transfer of weight over the standing leg.

Under normal circumstances the heel touches the floor first and the weight is transferred to the ball of the foot. But if the calf muscles become shortened the stretching that is necessary to allow the weight to move forwards over the foot cannot occur. The result is that the weight remains over the heel. If no adjustments are made the body will fall backwards. However, the body adjusts automatically by bending forwards at the hips to maintain balance.

This combination of a shortening of the calf muscles and bending forwards at the hips puts pressure on the large muscle which attaches above and below the knee to the Achilles tendon. Because this muscle passes across both the knee and ankle joints it will affect both joints if it becomes shortened. In severe cases it causes the foot to push downwards and the knee to become too straight.

The effect of bending forwards at the hips and the knee being pushed backwards is a severely distorted position when standing, and it is not uncommon for people to complain of pain in the knees because of this. This bending forwards at the hips also affects the upper body by putting additional strain on the lower back, which can cause problems in this area.

These are some of the ways in which the body compensates for the loss of range of movement in the foot and ankle. For the majority of people with CMT these compensations are preventable if action is taken early enough to stretch the most vulnerable muscles before they become shortened. **This stretching must only be carried out under guidance from a physiotherapist.**

Any attempt to stretch the muscles once they have shortened can cause problems in other areas. For example, if the foot is forced into a right angle position when the Achilles tendon has shortened, extra pressure will fall on the inner border of the foot. This can cause the arch to collapse, resulting in a flat and painful foot.

A person with CMT may find that their balance is also affected by the sensory loss caused by their condition. For example, many find it difficult to balance in bare feet. This is because, in addition to the muscles involved in maintaining balance, the body depends on sensory information from the feet to tell it what kind of surface it is standing on (carpet, hard floor, a slope, etc) and how it should adjust accordingly.

For these reasons a physiotherapist may prescribe insoles or splints to control the position of the feet and ankles when the muscle weakness affects walking. Many people dislike wearing these supports because they feel it is giving in to the condition, or because it makes them appear more disabled than they really are. In fact, the reverse is true: by keeping the feet in a better position the splints allow more normal activity throughout the rest of the body, which makes walking a much less strenuous activity.

Problems relating to hand function

The wasting of the small muscles in the hand is a characteristic of CMT. These muscles are used for the fine movements in activities such as writing, fastening and unfastening buttons, holding a knife and fork, and sewing. The problems arise from an inability to bring the thumb and index finger together.

The extent to which the hands can be affected varies considerably. Exercise to maintain the strength of these muscles is usually ineffective and overusing them can hasten the decline in function.

Secondary complications are less apparent and less severe than those arising from the weakness in the feet. As hand movements become more difficult problems may arise as a result of the increased use of the upper arms. People with more severe hand problems often complain of a feeling of tightness or strain across the neck and shoulders.

Advice should be sought from a physiotherapist or occupational therapist about aids and appliances that are available to make everyday tasks easier. These have been designed to replace the need for fine manual dexterity and strength and range from button hooks to electric can openers (see 'Aids to daily living' on page 75).

For example, when it is no longer possible to hold a pen correctly between the tips of the thumb and fingers, a special pen or thumb opposition splint may be beneficial. This will make tasks like writing less strenuous and perhaps even slow down the progressive weakness in the muscles. (A thumb opposition splint is a flexible, lightweight plastic mould which slips over the thumb and holds it in a position where it can easily touch the fingers. It can be slipped off when not required.)

Some simple exercises

The following are examples of exercises that might be of benefit to someone with CMT. The number of times each exercise is performed depends on the individual. 'A little and often' will be of greater benefit than prolonged exercise for any particular muscle. Tiredness is a recognised feature of CMT and over-exertion may be detrimental.

Note: Do not attempt any of the following exercises without first discussing them with a physiotherapist or your doctor, especially if you have had surgery to limit movement, such as a triple arthrodesis.

Foot exercises

- Stand facing a high table (a kitchen unit is ideal) with your hands on the surface. Keep your heels flat on the floor and lean forwards while keeping your knees and hips straight. Stop when you feel a stretch over the calf muscles. If there is sensory impairment be careful not to overstretch.

- Sit on a chair with your knees and ankles at right angles. Keep your heels on the floor while taking the knees forwards to increase the angle of bend at the ankle and knee.

Abdominal exercises

- Lie on a bed on your back with your knees bent and flatten the middle of your back into the bed. Lift your head and reach forwards to touch your knees with your hands. This will strengthen the abdominal muscles and thereby help to prevent increased curvature of the spine.

General exercises for ensuring correct body alignment

- Stand with your back to a wall with your feet positioned approximately an inch from it. Press your spine into the wall keeping your hips and knees straight. Try to shorten the distance between your tummy button and the nipple line. The shoulder girdles should remain in contact with the wall throughout.

- Sit on the edge of a table with your feet flat on the floor. Raise yourself into a standing position ensuring the knees first move forwards over the feet. Only straighten fully when the hips are straight. (Place a mirror to one side to help you assess this movement.)

Surgical procedures to correct problems with the feet

Many people have surgery on their feet to stabilise or correct the progressive problems which can arise from CMT, but it does not help everyone. The procedures range from straightening the toes, particularly the big toes, to fairly major surgery on the ankle joints.

There is no perfect time to have foot surgery as the recovery period is usually long. Neither is there an age limit for the operation, but at any age the inconvenience and risks of surgery must be balanced against the relief of pain and ease of walking.

Having the lower leg in plaster after surgery does not usually cause any specific problems as the foot muscles are not much used in walking. (It is true that there is some muscle loss while the leg is in plaster but it often does not affect walking ability afterwards. The gains of improved position and alignment usually outweigh the loss of muscle bulk and strength.)

Anyone who thinks they may need surgery should seek a referral through their family doctor or neurologist to an orthopaedic surgeon with a special interest in CMT.

CMT International UK's advice: If you have trouble finding an orthopaedic surgeon who is familiar with CMT we may be able to help you, but you may have to travel some distance for a consultation. If you decide to have surgery make sure you tell the anaesthetist that you have CMT. Some types of anaesthetic can cause problems, so the anaesthetist must be aware of your condition (see page 32).

The most common deformities with CMT

As CMT develops, the various muscles in the feet, and to a lesser extent the hands, are affected at different stages. This causes an imbalance in the way the feet look and perform, causing deformities of various kinds.

At first the deformity is flexible: ie, the foot can be pulled into a straight position even though it may revert to a deformed position when it is released. At this point the deformity is known as a correctable deformity. However, as time passes, the deformity becomes rigid and fixed and it is not possible to force the foot back into a 'normal' shape.

The common deformities are known as cavus and cavo-varus ('high arches'). The short flexor muscles and small intrinsic foot muscles tighten and contract and this causes high arches and clawing of the toes. Extensor weakness causes foot drop and club foot deformity. In the hands, intrinsic muscle weakness leads to hand muscle atrophy, extensor weakness and wrist drop.

The basic principles of managing the condition fall into three stages. Firstly, orthoses may be useful either to correct the deformity or to accommodate it. Splints may be used to correct mobile foot drop, ankle foot orthoses or callipers may correct mobile foot and ankle deformities, and surgical boots and inserts can be used to accommodate fixed deformities. However, there can be problems if the orthoses do not fit correctly and cause sores and rubbing which may go unnoticed if there is severe sensory loss.[16]

Secondly, soft tissue surgery may be used for correctable deformities, either to release contractures or to transfer tendons. As a final resort bone surgery can be performed to correct fixed deformities. Occasionally bone surgery may be performed alongside soft tissue procedures.

A brief description of some of the different operations follows. But note that some surgeons may use methods that differ from these.

---

16 Heavy metal callipers are rarely used nowadays since the additional strain of lifting them can actually cause a deterioration in the leg muscles. Ankle foot orthoses can help people who have major balance and fatigue problems. Made of plastic, they go under the foot and up the back of the leg, fastening around the leg with Velcro. Although they are lightweight, easy to wear and barely visible, these supports must be custom-made and fitted correctly. Ideally, they should not be worn for more than eight hours a day, since this could lead to major atrophying problems. For more information about orthoses see 'Some commonly asked questions about orthotics' on page 68.

Procedures to correct clawing of the toes

- **For a flexible deformity** – The correction can be achieved by taking a tendon from under the sole of the foot and transferring it to the top of the toes to help strengthen and thereby straighten them.

- **For a rigid deformity** – This can be corrected by interphalangeal fusion: ie, by removing the joint, straightening it and fixing it together with a pin.

- **In the big toe** – Interphalangeal fusion and tendon transfer (the 'Jones procedure') is performed.

Procedures to correct the cavo-varus foot

- **For a flexible deformity in children** – The plantar fascia ligament, which causes the high arch, is stripped from its attachment at the heel, effectively lengthening the ligament. The procedure is known as a plantar soft tissue release. It is not always a permanent solution and further surgery may be needed.

- **For a rigid arch with no inturning of the heel** – This can be corrected with a tarsal wedge osteotomy. This involves taking a wedge of bone from the middle of the foot, thereby lowering the arch and raising the foot.

- **For a rigid cavo-varus deformity (arch and heel deformity)** – This can be corrected, usually permanently, with a triple arthrodesis. This involves removing three sections of bone from the three joints in the heel and reconnecting them in the correct position with pins or staples to bring the foot into a more 'normal' shape. This can be an excellent long-term operation but it is never performed on children who are still growing because the sections that are removed are the growth plates on the heel joint and this would leave the child with a heel that does not grow.

Tendon transfer may be performed with a triple arthrodesis, either through the bony fusion mass or at the ankle joint, since the deformity may recur if the deforming tendon is not released.

Bone and tendon operations need to be protected carefully in plaster for up to 12 or more weeks after surgery because the stitches are not strong enough until the tissues have healed.

Procedures to correct foot drop

Orthoses may be sufficient when the foot drop can be corrected passively, or a tibialis posterior tendon transfer can be performed. This procedure releases the tendon which normally pulls the foot down into the deformed position and moves it through the leg to pull the foot upwards and outwards. Unfortunately the tendon does not always work so well after it has been moved.

For really serious foot drop a Lambrinudi triple arthrodesis can be performed. This involves cutting a number of bones in the foot and reassembling them to bring the foot to a 90 degree angle.

CMT International UK's advice: All types of surgery involve a trade-off between the potential benefits and a loss of muscle power and this should be considered very carefully before proceeding. Most tendon or bone surgery takes a long time to recover from, but if the procedures are skilfully performed in a specialist centre the outcome can be good.

Some commonly asked questions about orthotics

Q. What is an orthotist?

A. An orthotist is a designer of externally applied mechanical devices which can control, prevent or reduce the effects of the physical limitations of the body.

Q. What can an orthotist do for me?

A. People who are affected by CMT may have physical difficulties which limit their ability to walk efficiently. The severity of these difficulties can vary enormously from one individual to another, even within the same family. There are specific muscle groups affected by CMT which lead to the problems that are characteristic of the disease. These muscles have particular jobs, lifting the foot upwards and pulling the foot outwards. The orthotist is able to design a number of different splints to assist in controlling the foot and ankle, some of which are very simple while others are quite complex.

Q. Do I need to see an orthotist?

A. Your consultant neurologist or orthopaedic consultant will refer you to an orthotist if they feel it is necessary. You can also ask your family doctor to make a direct referral if you think it might help.

Q. I have seen an orthotist and the orthosis they provided just made me more uncomfortable. What should I do?

A. The types of orthoses which can help with CMT range from simple insoles and lightweight plastic splints to custom-made footwear and traditional metal callipers. The effects of CMT are so varied that the most appropriate orthosis will be different for everyone. It is the orthotist's job to determine which orthosis will work best for you and that it is as lightweight, comfortable and cosmetic as possible. If you are unhappy with the orthosis you should first complain to the orthotist. If you are still unhappy you can complain to the referring consultant or your family doctor.

Q. Will my orthosis make me better?

A. No. It should, however, make walking easier or more comfortable for you. It may also make the need for a corrective operation less likely.

Part 3
Practical issues

The addresses of all the organisations mentioned in this
section are listed in appendix 2

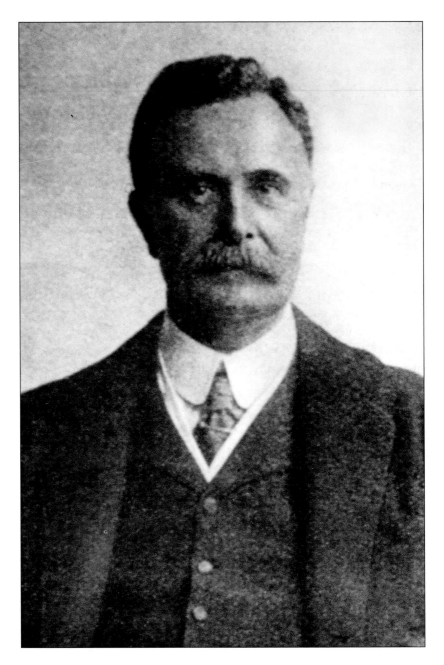

Plate III Howard Henry Tooth

Having a baby

Antenatal classes

Few antenatal staff know anything about CMT and many affected couples find that they spend their first few sessions at the antenatal clinic explaining the condition. CMT International UK can provide information leaflets that will help. The address is on page 87.

Pain relief during birth

Some women feel that delivery by caesarean section is the best option since it puts the least strain on the body. But there are alternatives: pethidine or gas and air (standard pain relievers) may be sufficient so that reserves of strength are intact when it comes to the actual delivery. An epidural painkiller, a spinal injection that kills all pain, **must** be discussed in advance with the anaesthetist who is to administer it. (For more about the important issue of CMT and anaesthesia see page 32.)

> **CMT International UK's advice:** Always be guided by the professionals but make sure they know about the implications of CMT and how it affects you. It is essential that they have all the information they need so they can advise you on the safest way of delivering your baby.

Prams and pushchairs

Manufacturers of prams, pushchairs, buggies, car seats and cots rarely seem to consider the problems of poor manual dexterity. Even the catches on drop-sided cots can be difficult.

CMT International UK's advice: Do not be afraid of going into your local mother-and-baby store and trying out all the catches, buckles and other mechanisms on the equipment you need. Ask for demonstrations of how pushchairs collapse and try all the buckles on car seats to be sure you can manage them. We suggest you do not buy large items on mail order unless you can first test them to your full satisfaction.

Useful sources of information

A good source of information on all aspects of pregnancy and parenthood is the National Childbirth Trust. Part of the Trust is the Disabled Parents' Network, a register of contacts who can provide support for parents with disabilities. All the people on the register receive a quarterly newsletter and a list of resources on a wide range of subjects.

Finding work and claiming benefits

There is plenty of evidence that unemployment rates are disproportionately high among disabled people and that it is more likely to be the result of discrimination than anything else.

The Disability Discrimination Act 1995 outlaws discrimination against disabled people in the workplace and requires employers to make reasonable adjustments for disabled employees, for example by designing a job around an individual, operating flexible hours, improving the physical environment, and so on. Note, however, that there are exemptions and that presently the law applies only to organisations with 15 or more employees.

Some employers display the Positive about Disability symbol (the 'two ticks' badge) on their advertisements. This means they have committed themselves to:

- interviewing all applicants with a disability who meet the minimum criteria for a job vacancy and considering them on their abilities

- discussing with disabled employees at least once a year how they can best develop and use their abilities

- making every effort to ensure disabled employees stay in employment

- taking action to ensure all employees develop disability awareness

- reviewing annually what has been achieved and informing employees and the Employment Service about the progress made.

CMT International UK's advice: If you are in work and the progressive nature of your CMT is making it difficult for you to cope, your employer may have a legal requirement to make reasonable adjustments to your working conditions or allow you to work reduced hours without loss of income. There are also schemes that provide equipment to enable you to work from home. It may not be necessary to give up work completely and a change of direction or retraining may be all that is required to find a job that is compatible with your degree of disability. It is always worth checking to see if something could be done to enable you to stay in work rather than feeling you just have to give it up.

Useful sources of information

The Disability Services Division of the Employment Service has its own disability employment advisers and runs a range of schemes, such as the Job Introduction Scheme, Access to Work and supported placement schemes, and produces a range of booklets and leaflets on all aspects of finding and keeping a job. These include *Make It Work* (DS2) and *Sources Of Information And Advice* (PGP6), both of which are available from Jobcentres or directly from the Disability Services Division of the Employment Service.

RADAR (the Royal Association for Disability and Rehabilitation) publishes a range of books, reports and information packs on a multitude of employment issues, including *Into Work*, which covers all aspects of working, interviewing skills, etc.[17]

Jobcentres have disability employment advisers who specialise in providing employment and training advice for people with disabilities.

The Department of Social Security provides a Freefone telephone number for people with disabilities who are seeking general advice and information on welfare benefits. The following leaflets are available from any local Social Security office: *Disability Living Allowance* (DS704), *Disability Living Allowance For Children* (DS706), *Attendance Allowance For People Over 65* (DS702), *Caring For Someone* (SD4), *Guide To Non-Contributory Benefits For Disabled People* (HB5), and *Incapacity Benefit (Sick Or Disabled)* (SD1).

---

17 RADAR is a national organisation run by and working for physically disabled people. It acts as a pressure group to improve the environment for disabled people, campaigns for their rights and needs and challenges negative attitudes and stereotypes. It is particularly involved with issues surrounding civil rights, social services, social security, employment, education, housing and mobility.

Aids to daily living

Adapting, altering or moving home

The design of many modern homes is very restrictive for people with any form of disability. Under the provisions of the Chronically Sick and Disabled Persons Act 1970 (see appendix 5) a person who has to adapt or alter their home because of the nature of their disability is entitled to an assessment of their housing needs by an appropriate professional (normally this would be an occupational therapist).

Local authorities have the discretion to award a number of means-tested grants to help with the cost of adaptations or alterations, the main ones being the Home Repair Assistance Grant (for adaptations valued at less than £1000) and the Disabled Facilities Grant. Details are available from the grants section of the environmental health department of every local authority. Smaller alterations and equipment may be available through the social services department (or its equivalent). Note that there can be variations in provision between England and Wales and Scotland and Northern Ireland.

If the home cannot be adequately altered or adapted the local authority may have an obligation to provide suitable alternative accommodation.

Home helps

People requiring assistance in and around the home may be eligible for help from the home care service, which is provided by the local authority. Referral to the service is usually through an occupational therapist and is dependent on an assessment of a person's needs and requirements.

The level of help available varies in different parts of the country and very much depends on the priorities within the area.

CMT International UK's advice: If personal care is required the home care service will probably be able to help. If you only require help with housework you may have some difficulty because, due to lack of resources, most home care services do not consider housework to be a priority.

Special aids and equipment

There are many companies providing special aids and equipment for people with disabilities. Most produce free catalogues. Two of the best are:

■ Keep Able Ltd, which runs a mail order service and has two stores in London and one in Brierley Hill in the West Midlands.

■ the Disability Equipment Register, which is the largest single source of used items of specialised disability equipment in the UK, Canada and North America.

The Disabled Living Centres Council is made up of a number of Disabled Living Centres where people with disabilities, their carers and people who work with or for them can inspect and try out a range of equipment designed to facilitate independent living. They give impartial and professional advice about the products best suited to an individual's needs and can provide information about all aspects of daily living for people with disabilities. A list of Disabled Living Centres may be obtained from the Disabled Living Centres Council.

CMT International UK's advice: We recommend sending off for the catalogues, deciding what you need, and then contacting your occupational therapist who may be able to provide the items free of charge or at a reduced cost.

Using a wheelchair

The vast majority of people with CMT will never need to use a wheelchair over the long term. However, even for occasional use wheelchairs can be invaluable (for making shopping trips easier, for example). Unfortunately, access to some places is still appalling, and if your arm muscles are not strong enough you will need someone to push. If you think you need a wheelchair you should speak to your doctor or occupational therapist who will make the necessary arrangements.

CMT International UK's advice: Do not think of using a wheelchair as giving up or giving in to the disease. Many people find that rather than restricting their movements the wheelchair gives them a means of continuing with activities which would otherwise have become impossible.

Useful sources of information

A list of housing associations catering for people with special needs is available from RADAR.

The Disabled Living Foundation can provide a wealth of information on many different subjects. Its publications include: *All Dressed Up* (a guide to choosing clothes and useful dressing techniques), *A Garden For You* (a practical guide to tools, equipment and garden design), and *With A Little Help* (a guide to equipment and services for independent living).

Driving with a disability

Driving licences for people with CMT

The Driver and Vehicle Licensing Agency's current rules on driving licences for people with CMT are set out in appendix 6.

The Mobility Advice and Vehicle Information Service

The Mobility Advice and Vehicle Information Service (MAVIS) was set up by the Department of Transport to help disabled and elderly motorists to make informed decisions about their own mobility needs. It provides practical advice on driving and vehicle adaptations and offers the opportunity to test drive a range of suitable vehicle types.

A disabled person can have their driving ability assessed by MAVIS. The assessment measures strength, steering force, reaction times, grip, seating position and other important factors. Assessment is by appointment only and there is a charge for the service.

Choosing a car

When choosing a car a person with a disability has the same basic requirements as anyone else – reliability, performance, comfort, appearance, cost – but the car must also be appropriate to their level of disability. Some of the considerations might be:

■ Does it need manual or automatic transmission? It is generally much less stressful for people with a disability to drive a car with automatic transmission, especially if they have weak upper limbs.

■ Does it need power-assisted steering? People with weak upper limbs are most likely to benefit from power-assisted steering.

■ Should it have two/three or four/five doors? A two/three door vehicle will generally have wider doors, which is particularly useful for transferring to and from a wheelchair.

- Should it be a hatchback, saloon or estate car? Drivers and passengers who use a powered wheelchair would need an estate car or a large hatchback to stow the wheelchair and would usually need some sort of hoist.

There may be additional considerations including:

- the ease of getting in and out of the car and the comfort of the seating
- the ease of operating the controls, including the secondary controls.

Motability

Motability is a hire purchase scheme which provides cars for recipients of the Disabled Living Allowance–High Rate Mobility Component (previously known as Mobility Allowance). In return for surrendering their allowance for four or five years the disabled person receives a car but must pay all maintenance and insurance costs themselves.

Alternatively, a car can be leased for a three-year period with all insurance and maintenance costs included. Under this option the driver is limited to 12000 miles per year.

Parking concessions for the disabled

The Orange Badge Scheme is a national arrangement of parking concessions for people with severe walking difficulties who travel either as drivers or passengers. It allows badge-holders to park closer to their destination but the national concessions apply only to on-street parking. There are some other benefits to having a badge but these can vary from area to area.

All new applications for an orange badge and all orange badges due for renewal after 1 April 2000 are to be replaced with the new European blue badge, which means all valid orange badges will have been replaced by 1 April 2003.

The new badge has been introduced to improve mobility opportunities for disabled people throughout the European Union. It means badge holders will be able to use the parking facilities for disabled people in each member state without the fear that their badge will not be recognised.

Further information is available from the Mobility Unit at the Department of the Environment, Transport and the Regions.

Useful sources of information

The Automobile Association (AA) and the Royal Automobile Club (RAC) both have schemes to help disabled drivers. The Disabled Drivers' Association and the Disabled Drivers' Motor Club are two organisations specifically for disabled drivers and produce a range of handbooks, journals and other information. Members of the Disabled Drivers' Motor Club benefit from a 15 per cent discount on most levels of RAC membership and discounts with many of the major ferry companies.

Door To Door: A Guide To Transport For People With Disabilities is a government publication covering all aspects of transport and is available from bookshops, libraries or direct from HMSO. RADAR's publications on the subject include *The Disabled Motorist* and *Motoring And Mobility For Disabled People*.

Leisure activities, holidays and travel

There are few, if any, leisure activities in which people with CMT cannot take part, including learning to fly (see below). Information on activities and classes is available from any local authority social services department or local disablement advice agency. Some useful national organisations are:

- Disability Sport England, which advises on different sports associations for disabled people

- the Riding for the Disabled Association, which provides a chance for people with any type of disability to go horse riding

- Gardens for the Disabled

- the National Listening Library, which loans books and cassettes

- PHAB England, a network of over 400 clubs (mostly youth clubs) where physically disabled and able-bodied people can mix socially on an equal basis.

People with almost any degree of disability can learn to fly. Flying Scholarships for the Disabled, a scheme set up in memory of the wartime pilot Douglas Bader, provides for up to ten disabled people a year to go to Atlanta, Georgia, for six weeks to learn to fly. To be successful, applicants must pass two days of medical examinations, interviews and aptitude tests.

Useful sources of information

Tripscope is a national travel and transport information and advice service for disabled and elderly people. It offers help with planning and organising journeys and can provide information on any travel-related problem. It is particularly helpful on travel insurance, since conditions like CMT may preclude normal insurance cover.

The Holiday Care Service publishes a booklet called *A Guide To Financial Help Towards The Cost Of A Holiday* which gives brief details of trusts and funds that offer financial help to disabled people.

RADAR has a wide range of booklets, fact sheets and access guides on holidays in

Britain, Europe, America and Australia. One of the best is *Access To Air Travel* which covers the whole process from booking a flight to making the airline aware of medical conditions, transporting wheelchairs and special equipment, insurance, and tips for first-time travellers.

Also available are: *Care In The Air: Advice For Disabled Travellers*, produced by the Air Transport Users' Committee, *Flying High: A Practical Guide To Air Travel* and *Personal Toilet On Long Flights*, from the Disabled Living Foundation.

Additional sources of help and assistance

Family care officers

The Muscular Dystrophy Campaign has a number of family care officers who could be of assistance in certain circumstances. Their job is to make sure that people have information about their condition and access to the services they need. They act as advocates for their clients – ie, someone who can speak out on their behalf, for example by writing letters or accompanying them to a hospital appointment – and offer psychological and moral support. For more information contact the Muscular Dystrophy Campaign.[18]

Contact a Family

Contact a Family was founded in 1979 with the aim of encouraging mutual support between families who have children with any type of disability or special need. It has a team of regional and national development officers who can offer advice on setting up parent support groups, and it publishes a range of fact sheets on topics such as special educational needs, benefits and holidays, and a quarterly newsletter, *Share An Idea*.

---

18 The Muscular Dystrophy Campaign is a UK charity which funds research into neuromuscular conditions and provides care and support for people who are affected by them. It also runs a neuromuscular centre in Cheshire, which provides training and employment for young people, and the Joseph Patrick Memorial Trust, an equipment fund.

Appendices

Appendix 1
About CMT International UK

CMT International is the support group for people with Charcot-Marie-Tooth disease, their carers and their families. It was founded in Canada in 1984 by Linda Crabtree, a journalist, who herself has CMT. By the time Linda held her first convention in 1986 she had made contact with over 700 people with the condition, mainly in North America.

CMT International UK was formed in 1986 and now has nearly 1000 members, mostly in the Home Counties, the Midlands and the north of England. Members receive a quarterly newsletter, *ComMenT*, and have the opportunity to attend the annual general meeting and conference, which is held in a different location every year.

In 1992 CMT International UK hosted the International Convention of CMT International in Stoke-on-Trent, the first time it had been held outside Canada. Fifty-nine delegates attended from all over Europe, Canada, the USA and Australia.

Much of the organisers' time is spent raising money to provide information resources for professionals, voluntary organisations and libraries and to help fund CMT-related research programmes under the auspices of the Muscular Dystrophy Campaign. The organisation also funds Outward Bound-type weekend breaks where younger members can take part in activities such as abseiling, yachting, swimming and horse riding.

CMT International UK is a registered charity, number 327971. Its patrons are Ms Julie Etchingham, the broadcaster, and Mr Jonathan Keeble, the actor.

For more information

Professional enquiries should be sent to:
Mrs Margaret Read
CMT International UK, 121 Lavernock Road, Penarth, South Wales CF64 3QG
Telephone 029 2070 9537
E-mail: mereadcmt@aol.com

Membership enquiries should be sent to:

Mrs Karen Butcher

CMT International UK, 36e Melbourne Road, Christchurch, Dorset BH23 2HZ

Telephone 01202 480285

E-mail: timkaren.butcher@ntlworld.com

CMT International UK also has a web site on the Internet at **www.cmt.org.uk**

Appendix 2

Addresses of useful organisations in the UK (as at June 2000)

from Part 1 CMT and anaesthesia

Medic Alert
1 Bridge Wharf, 156 Caledonia Road, London N1 9UU
Telephone 020 7833 3034

from Part 1 CMT and complementary medicine

The British Register of Complementary Practitioners
PO Box 194, London SE16 1QZ
Telephone 020 7237 5165

The Institute for Complementary Therapists
PO Box 194, London SE16 1QZ
Telephone 020 7237 5165

from Part 2 Coming to terms with CMT

The Association to Aid the Sexual and Personal Relationships of People with a Disability (SPOD)
286 Camden Road, London N7 OBL
Telephone 020 7700 0236

from Part 3 Having a baby

The National Childbirth Trust
Alexandra House, Oldham Terrace, Acton, London W3 6NH
Telephone 020 8992 8637

The Disabled Parents' Network
PO Box 5876, Towcester NN12 7ZN
Telephone 0870 241 0450

from Part 3 Finding work and claiming benefits

The Disability Services Division of the Employment Service
Rockingham House, 123 West Street, Sheffield S1 4ER
Telephone 08700 010171

The Royal Association for Disability and Rehabilitation (RADAR)
12 City Forum, 250 City Road, London EC1V 8AF
Telephone 020 7250 3222

The Department of Social Security
Freefone telephone number for people with disabilities: 0800 882200

from Part 3 Aids to daily living

Keep Able Ltd
Sterling Park, Pedmore Road, Brierley Hill, West Midlands DY5 1TB
Telephone 01384 484544

The Disability Equipment Register
4 Chatterton Road, Yate, Bristol BS37 4BJ
Telephone 01454 318818

The Disabled Living Centres Council
Redbank House, 4 St Chad's Street, Manchester M8 8QA
Telephone 0161 834 1044

The Disabled Living Foundation
380–384 Harrow Road, London W9 2HU
Telephone 020 7289 6111

from Part 3 Driving with a disability

The Mobility Advice and Vehicle Information Centre (MAVIS)
Macadam Avenue, Old Wokingham Road, Crowthorne, Berkshire RG45 6XD
Telephone 01344 661000

Motability
Goodman House, Station Approach, Harlow, Essex CM20 2ET
Telephone 01279 635666

The Mobility Unit, Department of the Environment, Transport and the Regions
Zone 1/11, Great Minster House, 76 Marsham Street, London SW1P 4DR
Telephone 020 7944 4140

The Automobile Association (AA)
Fanum House, Basingstoke, Hampshire RG21 2EA
Telephone 0800 262050

The Royal Automobile Club (RAC)
PO Box 700, Bradley Stoke, Bristol BS99 1RB
Telephone 0800 550550

The Disabled Drivers' Association
Ashwellthorpe, Norwich NR16 1EX
Telephone 01508 489449

The Disabled Drivers' Motor Club
Cottingham Way, Thrapston, Northamptonshire NN14 4PL
Telephone 01832 734724

Part 3 Leisure activities, holidays and travel

Disability Sport England
13 Brunswick Place, London N1 6DX
Telephone 020 7490 4919

The Riding for the Disabled Association
Lavinia Norfolk House, Avenue R, National Agricultural Centre, Stoneleigh Park, Warwickshire CV8 2LY
Telephone 024766 96510

Gardens for the Disabled

c/o Mrs F Seton, The Freight, Cranbrooke, Kent TN17 3PG

Telephone 01580 852249

The National Listening Library

12 Lant Street, London SE1 1QH

Telephone 020 7407 9417

PHAB England

Summit House, Wandle Road, Croydon, Surrey CR0 1DF

Telephone 020 8667 9443

Flying Scholarships for the Disabled

c/o The Principal, The Royal International Air Tattoo, Building 15, RAF Fairford, Gloucestershire GL7 4DL

Tripscope

The Vassall Centre, Gill Avenue, Bristol BS16 2QQ

Telephone 08457 585641

The Holiday Care Service

2nd Floor, Imperial Buildings, Victoria Road, Horley, Surrey RH6 7PZ

Telephone 01293 774535

The Air Transport Users' Committee

CAA House, 45–49 Kingsway, London WC2B 6TE

Telephone 020 7240 6061

from Part 3 Additional sources of help and assistance

The Muscular Dystrophy Campaign

7–11 Prescott Place, London SW4 6BS

Telephone 020 7720 8055

Contact a Family

170 Tottenham Court Road, London W1P 0HA

Telephone 020 7383 3555

Appendix 3

Clinical genetics centres in the UK

South East Thames Regional Genetics Service

Division of Medical and Molecular Genetics, 8th Floor Guy's Tower, Guy's Hospital, London SE1 9RT

Telephone 020 7955 4648

Catchment area: Lambeth, Southwark, Lewisham, Bromley, Greenwich, Bexley, Kent, East Sussex

South West Thames Regional Genetics Service

St George's Hospital Medical School, Cranmer Terrace, London SW17 0RE

Telephone 020 8767 8150

Catchment area: South-west London, Surrey, West Sussex

North East Thames Regional Genetics Service

Mothercare Unit of Clinical Genetics and Fetal Medicine, Institute of Child Health, 30 Guildford Street, London WC1N 1EH

Telephone 020 7242 9789

Catchment area: Enfield, Hampstead, Bloomsbury, Islington, Haringey, City and Hackney, Tower Hamlets, Newham, Waltham Forest, Redbridge, Basildon, Thurrock, Barking, Havering, Brentwood, Southend, North East Essex, Mid-Essex, West Essex

North Thames Regional Genetics Service

Clinical Genetics, Royal Free Hospital, Pond Street, London NW3 2QG

Telephone 020 7794 0500 extension 5163

Catchment area: Camden, New River, Edgware, Barnet, Newham, Whitechapel

North West Thames Regional Genetics Service

Kennedy Galton Centre, Northwick Park and St Marks NHS Trust, Watford Road, Harrow, Middlesex HA1 3UJ

Telephone 020 8869 2795

Catchment area: Barnet, Brent, Harrow, Hillingdon, Ealing, Hammersmith, Hounslow, Kensington, Chelsea, Westminster, Ashford, Hertfordshire, Bedfordshire

East Anglian Regional Genetics Service

Department of Clinical Genetics, Box 134, Addenbrooke's Hospital NHS Trust, Cambridge CB2 2QQ

Telephone 01223 331154

Catchment area: Hertfordshire, Bedfordshire, Lincolnshire, Cambridgeshire, Norfolk, Suffolk, North Essex

Oxford Regional Genetics Service

Department of Clinical Genetics, The Churchill Hospital, Old Road, Headington, Oxford OX3 7LJ

Telephone 01865 226000

Catchment area: Oxfordshire, Northamptonshire, Buckinghamshire, Berkshire, Swindon

Wessex Clinical Genetics Service

Princess Anne Hospital, Coxford Road, Southampton SO16 5YA

Telephone 023 8079 6166

Catchment area: Salisbury, Hampshire, Dorset, Isle of Wight

Clinical Genetics Service for Devon and Cornwall

Department of Child Health, Royal Devon and Exeter Hospital (Wonford), Exeter, Devon EX2 5DW

Telephone 01392 403151

Catchment area: Devon, Cornwall

Mersey Regional Genetics Service

Royal Liverpool Children's Hospital, Alder Hey, Eaton Road, Liverpool L12 2AP

Telephone 0151 228 4811

Catchment area: Liverpool, Wirral, Southport, St Helens, Knowsley, Warrington, Runcorn, Chester, Crewe, Isle of Man

Regional Clinical Genetics Service (Chester)

Moston Lodge, Countess of Chester Hospital, Liverpool Road, Chester CH2 1UL

Telephone 01244 364754

Catchment area: Chester, Warrington, Halton, Crewe, South Wirral

Department of Medical Genetics

St Mary's Hospital, Hathersage Road, Manchester M13 OJH

Telephone 0161 276 6262

Catchment area: Manchester, Oldham, Rochdale, Salford, Stockport, Tameside, Trafford, Wigan, Lancaster, Blackpool, Preston, Blackburn, Burnley, Chorley, Bolton, Bury

Clinical Genetics Unit

Institute of Child Health, Bristol Royal Hospital for Sick Children, St Michael's Hill, Bristol BS2 8BJ

Telephone 0117 928 5652

Catchment area: Avon, Somerset, Gloucester, Cheltenham

West Midlands Regional Clinical Genetics Service

Clinical Genetics Unit, Birmingham Maternity Hospital, Edgbaston, Birmingham B15 2TG

Telephone 0121 627 2630

Catchment area: Birmingham, West Midlands, Leicester, Staffordshire, Shropshire, Warwickshire, Hereford, Worcester

Yorkshire Regional Genetics Service

Department of Clinical Genetics, Ashley Wing, St James's University Hospital, Beckett Street, Leeds LS9 7TF

Telephone 0113 283 7070

Catchment area: Bradford, Leeds, Wakefield, Grimsby, Scunthorpe, North Yorkshire, West Yorkshire, East Riding

The Centre for Human Genetics

Langhill, 117 Manchester Road, Sheffield S10 5DN

Telephone 0114 271 7025

Catchment area: Sheffield, Barnsley, Doncaster, Worksop, Chesterfield, Rotherham, Buxton

Department of Clinical Genetics

2nd Floor H Block, City Hospital NHS Trust, Hucknall Road, Nottingham NG5 1PB

Telephone 0115 962 7711

Catchment area: Nottingham, North Nottinghamshire, South Derbyshire, North Derbyshire, Lincolnshire

Northern Region Genetics Service

19–20 Claremont Place, Newcastle upon Tyne NE2 4AA

Telephone 0191 222 7711

Catchment area: Cleveland, Durham, Tyne and Wear, Northumberland, Cumbria

Paediatric Genetics Unit

Royal Manchester Children's Hospital, Hospital Road, Pendlebury, Manchester M27 4HA

Telephone 0161 727 2335

Catchment area: Greater Manchester, Warrington, Lancashire, Cumbria

Leicestershire Clinical Genetics Service

Leicester Royal Infirmary, Leicester LE1 5WW

Telephone 0116 258 5736

Catchment area: Leicestershire

Northern Ireland Regional Genetics Service

Department of Medical Genetics, Floor A, Belfast City Hospital, Lisburn Road, Belfast BT9 7AB

Telephone 028 90 3555

Catchment area: Northern Ireland

Institute of Medical Genetics

University Hospital of Wales, Heath Park, Cardiff CF4 4XW

Telephone 029 2074 4028

Catchment area: Wales

West of Scotland Regional Genetics Service

Duncan Guthrie Institute of Medical Genetics, Yorkhill Hospital, Glasgow G3 8SJ

Telephone 0141 201 0365

Catchment area: Greater Glasgow, Argyll, Clyde, Ayrshire, Arran, Forth Valley, Lanarkshire, Dumfries, Galloway

South East Scotland Regional Genetics Centre

Department of Clinical Genetics, Western General Hospital, Crewe Road, Edinburgh EH4 2XU

Telephone 0131 651 1012

Catchment area: Lothian, Fife, Borders

Clinical Genetics Service

Department of Medical Genetics, Medical School, Foresterhill, Aberdeen AB9 2ZD

Telephone 01224 840749

Catchment area: Grampian, Highland, Orkney, Shetland, Western Isles

Cytogenetics Laboratory

Pathology Department, Royal Northern Infirmary, Ness Walk, Inverness IV3 5SF

Telephone 01463 704000 extension 3231

Catchment area: Highlands, West Grampian

Human Genetics Laboratories

Department of Pathology, Ninewells Hospital and Medical School,
Dundee DD1 9SY

Telephone 01382 632035

Catchment area: Dundee, Perth, North Fife, Angus, Perthshire

Appendix 4

Statutory assessment of special educational needs: A guide for parents

This section is intended to guide parents through the various stages of the statutory assessment of a child's special educational needs. Specific questions or queries should be discussed with the special needs staff at the local education authority.

The Education Act 1993 lays down procedures which a local education authority has to follow if a child is considered to have special educational needs which are so severe or complex as to require:

■ additional help at his or her primary or secondary school which cannot be provided from the school's normal resources

■ a placement at a special school or unit

■ the provision of education other than at school.

Identification and assessment

The local education authority must conduct a statutory assessment of the child's needs under section 167 of the Act. Normally a school-based or pre-school assessment will have been carried out by the school staff or pre-school advisory teacher, an educational psychologist or a support teacher for children with learning difficulties. The parents will have been consulted at that time.

When an authority proposes to make a statutory assessment of a child's special educational needs it must notify the parents of:

■ its proposal to make the assessment

■ the procedure to be followed

■ the name of the officer from whom further information may be obtained

■ their right to make representations and submit written evidence to the authority.

The next stage is for the parents to let the authority have:

■ their comments on the proposal to assess their child

■ any reports they have already obtained and would like to have included as part of the assessment

■ the names and addresses of any persons they would like the authority to consult in addition to those whom the authority must approach for educational, medical, psychological and social services advice

■ their views about their child's educational needs and what the authority should do to meet them.

A decision will then be made as to whether to proceed with a statutory assessment. If so, written advice will be sought from the child's school or pre-school advisory teacher, an educational psychologist, a medical officer and the social services department.

The child will usually be seen by an educational psychologist and a medical officer in the presence of the parents. (If the child has been seen only recently by the educational psychologist the parents may agree to waive this further assessment.)

The statement of educational needs

Once all the written contributions have been received the authority will consider whether the child's needs are severe enough to warrant a statement.

A draft statement will be issued summarising the child's needs and the provision the authority proposes to make to meet them – for example, additional teaching or non-teaching help within the local school or a placement at a school or school-based unit specialising in the education of children with special needs. At this stage the statement does not name the school; instead, the parents are invited to express a preference.

Parents have 15 days to respond to the draft statement. If they do not respond within this period the authority will assume they are happy with it and issue the final statement with the name of the school inserted. This document obliges the local education authority to make available to the child the educational provision specified.

Note in lieu of a statement

If the decision is not to issue a statement the education authority will instead issue a 'note in lieu of a statement'. This describes the child's special educational needs, includes all the submitted written advice, gives the reasons for not issuing a statement, and offers guidance as to how the child's needs can be met from the resources already at his or her school.

Timetable

The timetable for the statutory assessment process is as follows:

- **Considering whether a statutory assessment is necessary** – The period from the receipt of a request for a statutory assessment from the parents to the decision to make an assessment must be no more than six weeks.

- **Making the assessment** – The period from the education authority's decision to make an assessment to the decision to make a statement must be no more than ten weeks.

- **Drafting the statement or note in lieu of a statement** – The period from the education authority's decision to make a statement to the issuing of the draft statement or note in lieu of a statement must be no more than two weeks.

- **Finalising the statement** – The period from the issuing of the draft statement to the issuing of the final statement must be no more than eight weeks.

Guidelines for the parent's contribution to the statutory assessment

The assessment of a child's special educational needs is undertaken in partnership with the parents, who have a positive contribution to make to the final outcome. Copies of the parents' reports are sent to everyone who has been asked to contribute to the assessment.

The following headings are a guide to the areas parents may wish to think about when making their written contribution:

- What do you remember about your child's early years that might help? Were you happy about his or her progress? When did you first fear that things were not right? What is your child like now?

- General health and fitness, absences from school, serious illnesses or accidents, periods in hospital, tiredness

- Physical skills – walking, running, climbing, riding a bicycle, writing, etc

- Level of personal independence – dressing, coping with everyday routine, getting out and about

- What does he or she find easy or difficult?

- What do you think your child's special educational needs are? How do you think these needs can be best provided for?

- How do you compare your child with others of the same age?

- What is your child good at? What does he or she enjoy doing?

- What does your child worry about? Is he or she aware of the problem?

- What are your own worries and concerns?

Appendix 4a
Help with school examinations

Note: This section deals only with the special arrangements for GCSE examinations and is based on the personal experiences of one parent in one part of the country. It should not be taken as being representative of the situation in every part of the UK or for every type of exam.

Young people with CMT often find it difficult to write under exam conditions – ie, at speed and under pressure – at school or university. Special considerations can be made for candidates in the GCSE courses who have a permanent or long-term physical disability **providing they do not result in an unfair advantage over other candidates**. For people with CMT the special considerations are:

- **Additional time** – an additional allowance of up to 25 per cent of the total examination time can be allocated in most subjects at the discretion of the head of the examination centre except where the performance of a specific task in a limited time is an assessment objective.

- **Supervised breaks or rest periods** – either inside or outside the examination room. The duration of the break will not be deducted from the time allowed for the examination.

- **Use of special aids** – the candidate may use mechanical or technological aids and may dictate responses or have them transcribed.

- **Alternative accommodation** – examinations may be taken at home or in hospital, depending on the circumstances and at the discretion of the head of the centre.

An application for special arrangements must be made before 28 February in the year of the examination and may require the candidate to undergo additional medical, psychological and hearing tests, depending on the policy of the local education authority.

CMT International UK's advice: Each examination board and examination centre may have different rules for different types of examination. Parents should seek advice from their local education authority, or the university or other centre of higher or further education, as appropriate.

Appendix 5

Acts of Parliament relating to disabled people

The Chronically Sick and Disabled Persons Act 1970

Section 2 of this Act lists the various services that local authorities have a duty to provide if they consider a disabled person needs them. These are:

- practical help in the home (eg, a home help)

- a radio and/or television and assistance in using the local library

- lectures, games, outings and any help (including travel arrangements) needed to take advantage of educational facilities

- any adaptations such as a ramp or lift or special equipment needed for the greater safety, comfort or convenience of the disabled person

- holidays

- meals, either in the home or at a local centre

- a telephone and any special equipment needed to use it.

The Disabled Persons (Services, Consultation and Representation) Act 1986

This Act reinforces the duty of all local authorities to:

- assess a disabled person's need for services if asked to do so

- provide as much relevant additional information as possible

- take the abilities of carers into account when undertaking an assessment.

Section 4 of the Act reinforces the duty of local authorities to assess the needs of disabled people for any of the services listed in section 2 of the Chronically Sick and Disabled Persons Act 1970.

Section 8 requires local authorities when assessing needs to take into account the ability of a disabled person's carer to continue to provide care on a regular basis.

Section 9 requires social services departments to inform disabled people receiving any service from them of other relevant services provided by the local authority and any other authority or organisation.

The National Health Service and Community Care Act 1990

This Act contains provisions relating to the assessment of a disabled person's needs for community care. Section 47 of the Act requires local authorities to proceed as if the assessment were being carried out under section 4 of the Disabled Persons (Services, Consultation and Representation) Act 1986 without the disabled person having to request them to do so.

The Carers (Recognition and Services) Act 1995

Section 1 permits a carer as defined within the Act to request a local authority to consider the needs of the carer before making any decision under section 47 of the National Health Service and Community Care Act 1990.

The Disability Discrimination Act 1995

In July 1998 the government announced the implementation of part III of the Disability Discrimination Act 1995 which outlaws discrimination towards disabled people by any company, local authority or retail and entertainment outlet which provides goods, services or facilities to the general public. Since October 1999 organisations and companies have had a duty to review their policies, practices and procedures and to make 'reasonable adjustments' for disabled people. (What is considered 'reasonable' under the Act depends on the size, resources and nature of the organisation in question.) Regulations to make reasonable adjustments to make buildings physically accessible to disabled people will become law in 2004.

Rights and entitlements

The first step in obtaining any statutory service is to contact the local social services department and request an assessment of need. If the need for a service is recognised the social services department has a duty to arrange for it to be provided.

Note, however, that local authorities are entitled to recover the cost of any service they provide. Some apply a means test while others make an exemption for people who are receiving income support. What they **cannot** do is refuse or withdraw a service if the disabled person is unable to pay, although they have the right to try to recover the money through the courts as a civil debt.

It is also unlawful for a local authority to reduce or withdraw a service from someone unless his or her need for it has diminished.

Making a complaint about local authority services

The Local Authority Social Services Act 1970, section 7 (as amended by the National Health Service and Community Care Act 1990, section 50) requires local authorities to have in place a procedure for considering comments or complaints relating to the discharge of their duties. It also gives people the right to complain to the Secretary of State for Health if they feel their local authority has not fulfilled its duty towards them.

A copy of the complaints procedure should be available from any local authority social services department.

Appendix 6

Rules on driving licences for people with CMT

The rules on driving licences for people with CMT from the Driver and Vehicle Licensing Agency (DVLA) are often confusing and conflicting. CMT International UK asked the DVLA to provide definitive answers to some commonly asked questions.

Q. Is it true that the DVLA is becoming more selective on medical conditions and now allows some disabled drivers a driving licence up to the age of 70, or is it the case that once you have a three-year licence you must always have one? I used to have a three-year licence but I mislaid it and when it was replaced I was given a licence valid to the age of 70. Was this an error?

A. CMT must be notified to the Licensing Authority (Road Traffic Act 1988) because it is a condition which may affect safe driving. The DVLA considers each licence holder to be individually responsible for determining whether they have a disability which is relevant in terms of the law or one which, though not relevant at the moment, may give trouble in the future and would permit us within the terms of the Road Traffic Act to restrict the period of the licence.

We take the view that many people with CMT will not be unsafe, either now or in the future, and they therefore have a full licence. This explains why we may seem to do different things for different people. It also explains why it was not a mistake to issue the 'til 70' licence in the above instance. We have reviewed our policy and are prepared to give full 'til 70' licences to many people, not only those with CMT, where it seems they are unlikely to be a source of danger either now or in the future. Such people are of course obliged in law to notify the DVLA if there is an unfortunate and unpredicted relapse in their condition.

Q. If I do not disclose my CMT is the only offence I have committed one of making a fraudulent application? Presumably my licence is still valid and therefore the condition of my insurance that I must have a valid licence is not contravened.

A. A person who fails without reasonable excuse to notify the DVLA of a medical condition is guilty of an offence under the Road Traffic Act 1988, section 94(3), which could result in prosecution and a fine. Licence holders need to understand that many insurance companies take the view that insurance cover is rendered invalid if a medical condition is not declared both to themselves and to the DVLA.

Q. If I have a three-year licence must I pay a renewal fee unless I am receiving statutory benefits, in which case the fee will be reduced or waived?

A. There is no fee for medical renewal licences. However, there is a fee for renewals after the age of 70. This applies to everyone, whether they have a medical condition or not.

Appendix 7
The scientific history of CMT

Jean-Martin Charcot (1825–1893; see plate I) was the founder of modern neurology. A professor at the University of Paris, he opened what was to become the greatest neurological clinic of the time at the Saltpêtrière Hospital, which attracted students from all over the world, including Sigmund Freud. Charcot was the first to describe the disintegration of ligaments and joints caused by locomotor ataxia and related diseases. He also conducted pioneering research into identifying the sites in the brain responsible for specific nervous functions.

Pierre Marie (1853–1940; plate II) was a student of Charcot at the Saltpêtrière Hospital. His discovery that growth disorders are caused by pituitary disease contributed to the science of endocrinology. He also published the first description of acromegaly, a condition characterised by an overgrowth of bone tissue in the nose, jaw, fingers and toes, and traced the disease to a tumour of the pituitary gland at the base of the brain.

In 1886 Charcot and Marie collaborated on a scientific paper describing a form of progressive muscular atrophy they called the 'Charcot-Marie type'. At the same time a student at Cambridge University, Howard Henry Tooth (1856–1925; plate III), unaware of Charcot and Marie's work, published his doctoral thesis on the same subject. It was Tooth who suggested that peripheral nerve dysfunction caused the disease.

Important dates

1865	Virchow briefly describes the disease
1873	Friedreich describes some cases of progressive muscular atrophy
1886	Charcot and Marie, then Tooth, give a detailed description of the disease
1894	Marinesco reports anatomical findings in a case of Charcot-Marie
1905	Holmes describes combined CMT/spastic paraplegia
1926	Roussy and Levy report a particular form
1927	Davidenkow suggests a first classification
1956	Lambert demonstrates a slowing of the nerve conduction velocities
1957	Gilliatt and Thomas confirm Lambert's results

1958   Lambert *et al* describe heterogeneity in the slowing of nerve conduction velocities

1959   Gilliatt confirms the work of Lambert *et al*

1980   Bird *et al* suggest a localisation of CMT disease on chromosome 1 through linkage with the Duffy blood group

1983   Bird *et al* and Dyck present families not linked to chromosome 1

1986   Beckett suggests localisation Xp13 for X-linked dominant forms

1989   Vance *et al* suggest localisation of CMT disease on chromosome 1

1989   Haites *et al* confirm Beckett's work

1989   Raeymakers *et al* confirm the work of Vance *et al*

1991   Raeymakers *et al* and Patel *et al* discover duplication of chromosome 17 in patients with CMT disease

Acknowledgements

CMT International UK gratefully acknowledges the help given in the preparation of this book by all the contributors listed below, our medical advisers, and all past and present members of the executive committee.

The portraits of Jean-Martin Charcot and Pierre Marie are reproduced by kind permission of the Saltpêtrière Hospital, Paris.

Foreword

The Foreword is largely an adaptation of material which first appeared in the booklet *Coping With... Charcot-Marie-Tooth Disease* compiled and published by CMT International UK (revised edition 1997). Edited and reprinted with the permission of the publisher.

Material from *Coping With... Charcot-Marie-Tooth Disease* is also used in the following sections: 'How CMT is inherited' and 'CMT and complementary medicine' in Part 1, 'Tips for staying healthy' in Part 2, and 'Having a baby', 'Finding work and claiming benefits', 'Aids to daily living' and 'Leisure activities, holidays and travel' in Part 3.

Part 1 Genetic and medical issues

Part 1 is largely an adaptation of material which first appeared in *What Is Charcot-Marie-Tooth Disease?*, first published by CMT International UK in 1996 and revised in 1998 by Dr David Hilton-Jones MD FRCP FRCPE, and *Hereditary Motor And Sensory Neuropathies*, a fact sheet by Professor Anita Harding MD FRCP and Dr Hilton-Jones, published by the Muscular Dystrophy Group in 1998. Edited and reprinted with the permission of the publishers. Dr Hilton-Jones is a consultant neurologist at the Radcliffe Infirmary, Oxford. The late Professor Harding was professor of clinical neurology at the Institute of Neurology, London.

'The causes and symptoms of CMT' incorporates information on orthotics supplied by Gordon Steel, managing orthotist of the First British Orthotic Practice. This material is also used in 'Some commonly asked questions about orthotics' in Part 2.

'Prenatal testing for CMT type 1a' in the section 'How CMT is diagnosed' is an edited version of an article by Professor Harding which first appeared in *The CMTA Report*, the newsletter of the CMT Association in the USA. Edited and reprinted with the permission of the publisher.

'CMT and hereditary neuropathy with liability to pressure palsies' in the section 'CMT and some other conditions' is an edited version of an article by Maureen Horton, first published in *The CMTA Report* (Fall 1997). Edited and reprinted with the permission of the publisher.

'CMT and stress' by Linda Crabtree first appeared under the title 'Stress' in *The Mayo Clinic Health Letter* (December 1995). Material from 'Stress' is also used in the section 'Tips for staying healthy' in Part 2. Edited and reprinted with the permission of the author and the publisher. Linda Crabtree founded CMT International in Canada in 1984.

'CMT and anaesthesia' by Dr PJ Halsall and Professor FR Ellis of the Academic Unit of Anaesthesia at St James's University Hospital, Leeds, first appeared under the title 'Anaesthetics' in the Winter 1996 edition of *The Search*, the magazine of the Muscular Dystrophy Campaign. Edited and reprinted with the permission of the Muscular Dystrophy Campaign.

The glossary of scientific and medical terms was compiled by Professor Neva Haites, professor of medical genetics, University of Aberdeen.

Part 2 Living with CMT

'The impact of CMT on each stage of life' by Susan Salzberg first appeared under the title 'Child/youth developmental issues and CMT' in *The CMTA Report* (Summer 1992). Edited and reprinted with the permission of the author and the publisher. Susan Salzberg is an occupational therapist at the Durham VA Hospital, North Carolina.

'Coming to terms with CMT' by Patricia Dreibelbis first appeared under the title 'When a child is diagnosed' in *The CMTA Report* (Spring 1998). Edited and reprinted with the permission of the publisher.

'Tips for staying healthy' incorporates material from *Coping With... Charcot-Marie-Tooth Disease, Hereditary Motor And Sensory Neuropathies* (see above) and 'Preventing secondary complications' (see below).

'Hints on conserving energy' by Grace Young first appeared in *The CMTA Report*. Edited and reprinted with the permission of the publisher.

'Pain and pain control' by Linda Crabtree first appeared under the title 'Pain' in *The Canadian CMT International Newsletter* (June 1995). Edited and reprinted with the permission of the author and the publisher.

'Preventing secondary complications' was written specially for this book by Susan Edwards FCSP, formerly superintendent physiotherapist at the National Hospital, London.

'Surgical procedures to correct problems with the feet' was written specially for this book by Mr Paul Cooke ChM FRCS, consultant orthopaedic surgeon at the Nuffield Orthopaedic Centre, Oxford.

Part 3 Practical issues

'Finding work and claiming benefits' was written specially for this book by a former member of the executive committee of CMT International UK.

'Driving with a disability' by Ann Mells of the Mobility Advice and Vehicle Information Service (MAVIS) first appeared in *The PHAB Magazine* (Summer 1995). Edited and reprinted with the permission of the publisher.

Appendices

'Statutory assessment of special educational needs: A guide for parents' (appendix 4) is adapted from a leaflet issued by Devon County Council and is edited and reprinted with their permission.

'Help with school examinations' (appendix 4a) was written specially for this book by a former member of the executive committee of CMT International UK.

'Acts of Parliament relating to disabled people' (appendix 5) originally appeared as 'The Chronically Sick and Disabled Persons Act 1970' in *The RADAR Bulletin* (July 1998). Edited and reprinted with the permission of the publisher.

The answers to the questions in 'Rules on driving licences for people with CMT' (appendix 6) were provided by Dr Elizabeth Rowse MB MRCP(UK), senior medical adviser to the Driver and Vehicle Licensing Agency.

'The scientific history of CMT' (appendix 7) was compiled from a variety of sources including the *Encyclopaedia Britannica* and the *Journal Of The History Of The Neurosciences* (1992).